PRINCIPLES & PRACTICE OF ICD-10 CODING

Dhirendra Verma, M.S., Ph.D.
(Director General, Dayanand Dinanath Group of Institutions, Kanpur, India)

Ali Mohamed El-Sayed, M.P.H., M.D.
(Consultant, Dept. of Statistics & Medical Records, Ministry of Health, Kuwait)

ISBN 978-81-903812-2-2

First Edition: 2008, Second Edition : 2009 Rs. 395/-

 **ROCHAK PUBLISHING**

4/2 B, L.I.G. Govindpur Colony,
Allahabad-211004 (U.P.) India
Tel. (91) 09415091004
E-mail: editormuses@yahoo.com

Printed in India at Astha Associates, Allahabad

Contents

Contents

PREFACE

The traditional emphasis in medical records management around the world has been on *what* data to get, and not on *how* to get it. The more efficient health information systems of today, however, are interested in what data to get, how to get it, and how to synthesize these data into an understanding of the patient's total situation. Disease classification and coding is the principal tool used by medical records personnel to accomplish this, and is, therefore a skill, which the effective healthcare managers, medical records administrators, clinical statisticians, statistical technicians, and medical transcriptionists also must master. This book is designed to present the principles that will help the learner to acquire or improve that skill.

The roots of the book go back to the teaching of ICD coding to doctors, medical records personnel and statistical technicians at the Department of Statistics & Medical Records, Ministry of Health, Kuwait for over two decades. While teaching the principles and techniques of disease coding through various revisions of the ICD we came across many areas which were not within easy reach of our students, leading to frustration among them. This led us to bring out this comprehensive guidebook on ICD-10 coding with detailed explanations, suitable examples and appropriate coding exercises for better comprehension.

The book is divided into eight units. Unit 1 provides an introduction to disease coding. Unit 2 gives a brief history of the development of ICD Units 3 and 4 deal with the main classification and alphabetic index of ICD-10. Unit 5 explains the principles and techniques of using ICD-10 and Unit 6 does this on a chapter-by-chapter basis. Units 7 and 8 consider the special features of morbidity and mortality coding. Unit 9 emphasizes the various aspects of statistical presentation in accordance with the WHO regulations. Care has been taken all through these units to keep the matter as simple as possible. Appropriate examples are provided wherever needed. Suitable exercises are presented at the end of each unit, which the students can take to test their level of comprehension before embarking on to the next unit.

Many people have contributed to this final product. Of these, special mention should be made of Dr. Abdul Aziz Khalaf, Director of Statistics & Medical Records Department at the Ministry of Health, Kuwait for his continuous support and encouragement. We are deeply indebted to Miss Zahra Awadh who reviewe d most of the chapters and made many helpful contributions to both style and content; and to Mr. Mohamed Bader and Mrs. Jaya Umaputhiran for secretarial assistance.

We are especially grateful to hundreds of doctors, medical records administrators and technicians, health statisticians, and ICD coders who participated in our training programmes and workshops on ICD in Kuwait and other countries during the past 25 years. We trust that these many colleagues will find our account of some small value.

April, 2008

Dhirendra Verma
Ali M. El-Sayed

UNIT 1
INTRODUCTION TO DISEASE CODING

UNIT I

INTRODUCTION TO DISEASE CODING

Need for disease coding

When any substantial volume of data has to be recorded, a system of classification[1] and coding is necessary, and coding is especially important if the data are to be retrieved or analyzed by mechanical or electronic means. In the study of illness and death, therefore, a standard classification of diseases and injuries is essential in order to provide appropriate codes to various diagnostic statements recorded by physicians in the course of treating their patients.

Uses of disease coding

Disease coding is used for variety of purposes, but the two principal ones are to:

      i)   Assist record retrieval, and
      ii)   Produce statistics.

i)   **Record retrieval** is facilitated by accurate and detailed coding, allowing cases to be identified that fulfil specific disease criteria. An example would be *hypertensive renal disease*. Suitable coding would allow all relevant cases of this condition to be identified quickly and effectively.

ii)   For **statistical purpose**, diagnostic coding enables groups of diseases that have considerable affinity to be brought together to facilitate the deduction of general principles, and

---

[1]*A Classification is an orderly arrangement of objects or individuals into groups on the basis of certain common characteristics.*

to present their incidence and prevalence in society in a meaningful way. Statistics thus generated contributes to better management of health care.

Medical statistics are used to meet the varied requirements of clinics & hospitals, offices of vital & health statistics, medical records offices, social welfare and insurance organizations, health surveys, World Health Organization, and numerous other agencies.

The role of ICD in disease coding

The ICD (or International Classification of Diseases) is a statistical classification of diseases, injuries, and causes of death. Produced by the WHO (World Health Organization), it has been developing for more than 100 years as a systematic coding system. It allows a unique code to be assigned to any disease or condition diagnosed by physicians or other authorized health care practitioners. These codes are designed to be used for statistical purposes.

The ICD is an international classification and is designed to enable consistency of coding throughout the world. It is detailed and thorough enough for every possible disease and injury to have a place somewhere within the classification. Consistent use of ICD codes allows comparative statistics to be produced among hospitals, regions and nations.

Utility of ICD codes

ICD codes are utilized for morbidity and mortality coding. They are assigned using two main sources of information:

1.   **Morbidity**: - The sources of information relate to contacts with health services. For the coder they are usually medical records in hospitals and primary health care centres.

2.   **Mortality**: - The codes are assigned from registrations of deaths. Morbidity and mortality statistics are prepared for two main reasons
   a)   Epidemiology
   b)   Medical care management.

a) **Epidemiology**: - Epidemiology may be defined as *the study of the distribution and determinants of disease frequency (in man)*. It involves relating diseases and injuries to characteristics of the person, such as:
   - Age
   - Gender
   - Marital status
   - Area of residence
   - Occupation
   - Exposure to hazards
   - Social habits
And, in the newborn,

   - Birth weight
   - Length of gestation
   - Type of delivery

b) **Medical care management**: - Medical care management means knowing *how many people with each condition are attending for treatment*, and needs to relate the disease and injuries to such facts as:
   - Number with the disease or condition
   - Length of stay in hospital
   - Source of admission
   - Services consumed
   - Outcome of care

- Quality of care
- Cost of care

Medical care management is of increasing importance today as the overall cost of medical care tends to consume an ever increasing proportion of a country's wealth.

To summarize: If you think about the vast number of diseases which exist and the management activities that take place for their prevention and treatment, it would become obvious that routine statistics could not present figures about each individual disease in random order. Therefore, diseases have to be *arranged* in an orderly fashion, *grouped* to provide meaning, and *numbered* or *coded* so that the codes could be easily processed. *ICD is designed to carry out these functions.*

Exercise 1. Fill in the blanks to make the sentences complete:

1. ICD is an abbreviation for International
....
of ....

2. The initials W.H.O. stand for:

....

3. Diagnostic coding is used to assist record retrieval and produce
....

4. The two main reasons for which mortality & morbidity statistics are colleted, are: ....
and............................

5. .... is the study of the distribution and determinants of disease frequency.

6. The three epidemiological characteristics of the newborn on which it is important to collect statistics, are:

....

....

....

7. A classification is an orderly .... of objects or individuals into .... on the basis of certain common characteristics.

UNIT 2
HISTORY OF THE DEVELOPMENT OF ICD-10

UNIT 2
HISTORY OF THE DEVELOPMENT OF ICD-10*

Introduction

A classification of diseases may be defined as a system of categories to which morbid entities are assigned to established criteria. There are many possible axes of classification and the one selected will depend upon the use to be made of the statistics to be compiled. A statistical classification of diseases must encompass the entire range of morbid conditions within a manageable number of categories.

ICD-10, the full title of which is **"the International Statistical Classification of Diseases and Related Health problems--Tenth Revision"**, has a long but interesting history. The first known classification of diseases dates back to the year 1700, when the King of England charged his deputy, John Graunt, to estimate the proportion of live born children who died before the age of six years. This attempt resulted in the *London Bills of Mortality*, which listed 13 classes of disease in young children. It also helped him to estimate that 36% of the children in London died before the age of six.

In the same century, Francois Lacroix published his *Nosologia Methodica* (1750), the first systematic classification of diseases, and William Cullen of Edinburgh later published a similar work entitled *Synopsis Nosologia Methodicae* (1785).

---

* Most of the material presented in this chapter is based on the historical account provided in the 2nd Volume of ICD-10 (Second Edition), W.H.O., Geneva.

By the year 1853, the need for an international classification of diseases was recognized and the First International Statistical Congress was convened in Brussels. The prime mover was Dr. William Farr, Registrar General and Medical Statistician for England & Wales. All diseases were classified in 139 separate groups under five general headings. Statistics were needed for causes of death and for public health control especially because of contagious diseases. There was a particular need and a statistical classification was created to satisfy this need. This classification was revised at least three times.

ICD-1 to ICD-9

In 1893, Dr. Jacques Bertillon, the Chief Statistician for the city of Paris advanced a more detailed and well-organized classification and which may well be regarded as the first ICD.[1] Bertillon's Classification or *International List of Causes of Death* was adopted by many countries and was, eventually in 1928 and 1938, published by the Health Organization of the League of Nations.

In 1946, the World Health Organization (WHO) accepted responsibility for all subsequent revisions. In 1948 an important step was taken. The Sixth Revision Conference approved a comprehensive list for both mortality and morbidity, agreed on international rules for selecting the underlying cause of death, and adopted a program of international cooperation in the field of vital and health statistics. The publication title was also changed to *Manual of the International Statistical Classification of Diseases, Inquiries, and Causes of Death* and referred to as the *International Classification of Diseases, Sixth Revision* (ICD-6).[2]

---

[1] Bertillon, J. (1912), Classification of the Causes of Death, abstracted. *Trans. 15th Int. Cong. Hyg. Demog.* (Washington, D. C.)
[2] W.H.O. (1948), *Manual of the International Classification of Diseases, Injuries, and Causes of Death, 6th Revision*, Geneva.

Revision was accomplished and finally published in 1969; and in 1977, WHO published the Ninth Revision of this statistical classification, referred to as ICD-9.[3] All these revisions were published in two volumes. The first volume was a listing of classification categories with special tabulation lists for international reporting of causes of death. Volume II was an alphabetical index to the first volume.

A number of major changes took place with the Ninth Revision; some of the most innovative of them are listed below:[4]

- An optional fifth digit for certain codes to allow more specific coding.
- An independent optional classification for classifying the morphology of neoplasms (the M-codes).
- An optional dual code for etiology & manifestation (the dagger & asterisk code) of disease conditions.
- A comprehensive glossary for mental disorders.

ICD-10

Work on the Tenth Revision of the ICD started in September 1983, when a Preparatory Meeting on ICD-10 was convened in Geneva. The programme of work was guided by regular meeting of Heads of WHO Collaborating Centres for Classification of Diseases. Policy guidance was provided by a number of special meetings including those of the Expert Committee on the International Classification of Diseases – Tenth Revision, held in 1984 and 1987.

---

[3] W.H.O. (1977) *Manual of the International Statistical Classification of Diseases, Injuries, and Causes of Death, 9th Revision*, Geneva.

[4] See also Appendix – "B"

In addition to the technical contributions provided by many specialist groups and individual experts, a large number of comments and suggestions were received from WHO Collaborating Centres for Classification of Diseases [5] as a result of the global circulation of draft proposals for revision in 1984 and 1986. From the comments received, it was clear that many users wished the ICD to encompass types of data other than the 'diagnostic information' (in the broadest sense of the term) that it has always covered. In order to accommodate the perceived needs of these users, the concept arose of a 'family'[6] of classifications centred on the traditional ICD with its familiar form and structure. The ICD itself would thus meet the requirement for diagnostic information for general purposes, while a variety of other classifications would be used in conjunction with it and would deal either with different approaches to the same information or with different information (notably medical and surgical procedures and disablement).

Following suggestions at the time of development of the Ninth Revision of the classification that a different basic structure might better serve the needs of the many and varied users, several alternative models were evaluated. It became clear, however, that the traditional single-variable-axis design of the classification, and other aspects of its structure that gave emphasis to conditions that were frequent, costly or otherwise of public health importance, had withstood the test of time and that many users would be unhappy with any of the models that had been proposed as a possible replacement. Consequently, as the study of the Tenth Revision will show, the traditional ICD structure has been retained but an alphanumeric coding scheme replaces the previous numeric one.

---

[5] See Appendix – "A" for a complete list of all ICD collaborating centres of the WHO.

[6] See Appendix – "C" for the WHO Family of International Classifications (WHO-FIC)

This provides a larger coding frame and leaves room for future revision without disruption of the numbering system, as has occurred at previous revisions.

One of ICD-10's most innovative features is the establishment of an updating process within the ten-year revision cycle. Thus the Second Edition of ICD-10 was brought about in 2004. It included the corrigenda to Volume 1, which appeared as an addendum to Volume 3 of the First Edition, as well as the updates that came into effect between 1998 and 2003.

In order to make optimum use of the available space, certain disorders of the immune mechanism are now included with diseases of the blood and blood-forming organs (Chapter III). New chapters have been created for diseases of the eye and adnexa and diseases of the ear and mastoid process. The former supplementary classifications of external causes and of factors influencing health status and contact with health services now form part of the main classification.

The dagger and asterisk system of dual classification for certain diagnostic statements, introduced in the Ninth Revision, has been retained and extended, with the asterisk axis being contained in homogeneous categories at the three-character level.

Contents of the three volumes of ICD-10

The presentation of the classification has been changed and there are now three volumes:

Volume 1. **Tabular List.** This contains the Report of the International Conference for the Tenth Revision, the classification itself at the three-and four-character levels, the classification of the morphology of neoplasms; special tabulation lists for mortality and morbidity, definitions, and the nomenclature regulations.

Volume 2. **Instruction Manual.** This brings together the notes on certification and classification formerly included in Volume 1 with a good deal of new background and instructional matter and guidance on the use of Volume 1, on tabulations, and on planning for the use of ICD, which was seen as lacking in earlier revisions. It also includes the historical material formerly presented in the introduction to Volume 1.

Volume 3. **Alphabetical Index.** This presents the index itself with an introduction and expanded instructions on its use.

The next two units deal with the structure and layout of Volume 1 (The Main Classification) and Volume 3 (Index) in greater detail.

Exercise 2 Circle either T (True) or F (False) where appropriate:

1. The full title of ICD-10 is "The International Classification of Diseases -- Tenth Revision".	T	F
2. The first known classification of diseases goes back to the Year 1800.	T	F
3. The author of the *London Bills of Mortality* was Dr. John Graunt.	T	F
4. Dr. William Farr, in 1853, classified all known diseases Into 139 separate groups under 5 general headings.	T	F
5. "Classification of Causes of Death" was advanced by Dr. Jacques Bertillon in 1893.	T	F
6. ICD-7 was published in 1975.	T	F
7. The Dagger & Asterisk Classification was introduced in ICD-8.	T	F
8. A comprehensive glossary for mental disorders was provided in ICD-9.	T	F
9. ICD-10 was published in 1990.	T	F
10. ICD-10 can be updated *within* the ten-year revision cycle.	T	F

UNIT 3
THE MAIN CLASSIFICATION (VOLUME 1)

UNIT 3

THE MAIN CLASSIFICATION (VOLUME 1)

Introduction

Most of Volume 1 is taken up with the main classification, composed of the list of three-character categories and the tabular list of inclusions and four-character subcategories. The former (i.e. the list of three-character categories) is the required or mandatory level for reporting to the WHO mortality database and for general international comparisons. In addition, Volume 1 also contains the following, which are to be found at the end of the volume.

(i) Morphology of neoplasms

The classification of morphology of neoplasms may be used, if desired, as an additional code to classify the morphological type for neoplasms, which are classified in Chapter II only according to behaviour and site (topography).

(ii) Special tabulation lists

Because the full four-character list of the ICD, and even the three-character list, are too long to be presented in every statistical table, most routine statistics use a tabulation list that emphasizes certain single conditions and groups others. The four special lists for the tabulation of mortality are an integral part of the ICD. Lists 1 and 2 are for general mortality and lists 3 and 4 are for infant and child mortality (ages 0-4 years). There is also a special tabulation list for morbidity.

(iii) Definitions

The definitions in Volume 1 have been adopted by the World Health Assembly and are included to facilitate the international comparability of data.

(iv) Nomenclature regulations

The regulations adopted by the World Health Assembly set out the formal responsibilities of WHO Member States regarding the classification of diseases and causes of death, and the compilation and publication of statistics.

Arrangement of the Main Classification

The main classification is divided into 22 chapters, marked by Roman numerals. Chapters I to XVII relate to diseases and other morbid conditions, and Chapter XIX to injuries, poisoning and certain other consequences of external causes. The remaining chapters complete the range of subject matter nowadays included in diagnostic data. Chapter XVIII covers symptoms, signs and abnormal clinical and laboratory findings, not elsewhere classified, and Chapter XX lists the External Causes of morbidity and mortality.

Chapter XXI (Factors influencing health status and contact with health services) is intended for the classification of data explaining the reason for contact with health care services of a person not currently sick, or the circumstances in which the patient is receiving care at that particular time or otherwise having some bearing on that person's care.

Chapter XXII (Codes for special purposes) is a new addition to the Second Edition of the ICD-10, which makes use of the letter U that was formerly set aside for the provisional assignment of new diseases of uncertain etiology or for research use when testing an alternative sub-classification for a special project. At present this chapter contains only one block but would contain many more in future additions of ICD-10.

Types of Chapters

ICD-10 groups diseases in a combination of ways: some based on types of diseases, some on parts of the body and some on external factors. There are two types of chapters – "Body Systems" chapters and "Special Groups" chapters. A disease of the "body system" is one, which would only affect a particular part of the body (e.g. Chapter XI, Diseases of the *digestive system*). Chapters VI – XIV are considered the "Body Systems" chapters. In "Special Groups" chapters, the diseases are linked by some factors other than the part of the body. They may not be restricted to a particular part of the body or body system and may affect the entire body. An example might be an infectious disease such as measles. While the symptoms of measles manifest in specific parts of the body (such as the skin and eyes), the disease itself is placed in a "Special Groups" chapter containing most of the infectious diseases (i.e. Chapter I, Certain infectious & parasitic diseases). Chapters I-V, XV-XVII, XIX and XXII are "Special Groups" chapters. Chapter XVIII is considered a "General" chapter as it contains general conditions that are not well defined such as symptoms, signs, etc. (e.g. headache, cough, fatigue, pain).

Chapters XX and XXI are regarded as "External Factors" chapters. Comments in case notes, which refer to external factors, are easily recognized. Here are some examples: *fall from ladder, drug poisoning, routine antenatal checks, and immunization.*

Exercise 3.1 Which chapters in the following table are assigned over to diseases of the body systems, which to special diseases, which to external factors, and which to general conditions? (Mark by placing B, S, E or G against the chapter:

CHAPTER	MARK	CHAPTER	MARK
" I		" XII	
" II		" XIII	
" III		" XIV	
" IV		" XV	
" V		" XVI	
" VI		" XVII	
" VII		" XVIII	
" VIII		" XIX	
" IX		" XX	
" X		" XXI	
" XI		" XXII	

Principles Governing the Choice of a Chapter

The distinction among the various types of chapters has practical implications for understanding the structure of the classification, for coding to it and for interpreting statistics based on it. Two general principles govern the choice:

i) The "Special Groups" chapters have priority over the "Body Systems" chapters. Thus, "Neoplasm of lung" would be coded from Chapter II (Neoplasms) and not from Chapter X (Diseases of the Respiratory System). Likewise, "Dementia", a brain disorder, finds a place in chapter V (Mental & Behavioral Disorders) and not in chapter VI (Diseases of the Nervous System).

i) Both, the "Special Groups" chapters and the "Body Systems" chapters have priority over the "General" chapter (i.e. Chapter XVIII). Chapter XVIII is to be used when a diagnosis simply cannot be coded more specifically from any of the other chapters. Thus "Abdominal and pelvic pain" could only be assigned a code R10 from Chapter XVIII (R10) if not found to be related to a more specific cause such as "renal colic" (N23, Diseases of the genitourinary system, Chapter XIV), "Pylorospasm" (K31.3, Diseases of the digestive system, Chapter XI), or "Dorsalgia" (M54, Diseases of the musculoskeletal system, Chapter XIII).

Exercise 3.2

> Which of the following cases should be classified as a special disease and which as a disease of a body system? Mark it by 'S' or 'B'
>
> 1. ASTHMA.
>
> 2. STOMACH ULCER.
>
> 3. LEUKEMIA.
>
> 4. KIDNEY STONE.
>
> 5. HYPERTENSION COMPLICATING PREGNANCY.
>
> 6. CHOLERA.

The chapters represent the first level of classification in ICD-10. This is the first point at which diagnoses are allocated to a specific area of the classification. The title of the chapter describes the specific contents of the chapter and is followed by the chapter number. The range of codes that a chapter may have is shown in parentheses following the title, e.g. Chapter II, Neoplasms (C00 – D48).

Usually a chapter is associated with one letter of the alphabet for all codes within it. However, some large chapters use more than one letter for their codes. Thus Chapters I, II, and XIX each have two letters assigned to them (A &B, C&D, S&T, respectively) and Chapter XX as many as four (V, W, X, Y). On the other hand, some letters are used for more than one chapter. For example, the letter D is used in both chapters II (Neoplasms), and Chapter III (Diseases of the blood & blood-forming organs). Another example is letter H, which is used in both Chapter VII (Diseases of the eye and adnexa), and Chapter VIII (Diseases of the ear and mastoid process).

There is enough provision in each chapter to cover its contents. Almost each chapter has a number of categories, which have not been used. This has been done to allow sufficient space for future revision and expansion. To illustrate, Chapter III (Diseases of the blood & blood-forming organs) has been assigned 40 categories (D50-D89), out of which only 34 are actually used, leaving six (D54, D78, D79, D85, D87 and D88), for future use. What's more, 10 more categories are readily available (D90-D99), should there be a need for more diseases of blood & blood-forming organs to be classified in the near future.

Specific chapter notes

In some chapters where it is felt that the coder may experience some difficulty in coding properly, explanatory notes are provided to simplify things.

Chapter II (Neoplasms) is an example where a set of such notes (# 1 to 8), could be found at the beginning of the chapter.

Inclusion and exclusion terms

At the beginning of each chapter, there are listed a number of "inclusion" and "exclusion" terms, as examples of the diagnostic statements which are "included" in, or "excluded" from that particular chapter. These terms are listed as a guide to the contents of the chapter and the coder must pay attention to them prior to assigning a code for a diagnostic statement from that chapter. A good example is Chapter V (Mental and behavioural disorders) where these two terms are listed right under the chapter title in the form of two statements -- *Includes:* disorders of psychological development, and *Excludes:* symptoms, signs and abnormal clinical and laboratory findings, NEC (R00-R99).

What it means is that this chapter *includes* codes for only those mental and behavioural disorders that are of psychological development, and are well defined, clinically recognized diseases of the mind such as schizophrenia, dementia, personality disorders, and various types of neuroses and psychoses. However, it *excludes* those conditions that may look like mental and behavioural disorders but are ill-defined and don't have a demonstrable etiology in cerebral disease, brain injury or other insult leading to cerebral dysfunction. Some examples of such conditions are: nervousness, disorientation, amnesia, suicidal tendencies, and hallucinations. Such "excluded" conditions may be coded from another chapter and the coder is explicitly guided to that chapter. For example, the notation *Excludes* at the beginning of chapter V clearly indicates (in parentheses) the chapter and codes where such conditions are classified (i.e. R00-R99).

Inclusion and Exclusion terms are not limited only at the chapter level, they are found at the category level as well. For example, category K44, Diaphragmatic hernia (chapter XI, Diseases of the digestive system) *includes* only this type of developmental hernia, which is also commonly known as hiatus hernia or paraoesophageal hernia. But it *excludes* such type of hernia if it is congenital in nature. In that case, it should be looked at elsewhere, and to assist the coder, even the appropriate codes are provided, in parentheses (i.e. Q79.0, Q40.1), at the end of the exclusion statement.

Exercise 3.3

Look at Chapter I and answer the following questions:

a) What is "included" exactly in this chapter?

....

b) What respiratory infections are "excluded" from this chapter?

....

c) Where can we find the exact codes for these "excluded" respiratory

   infections?

....

d) Can you find an example of both, inclusion and exclusion, terms in

   Chapter I at the category level?

....

Conventions

In listing inclusion and exclusion terms in the tabular list, the ICD employs some special conventions relating to the use of parentheses, square brackets, colons, the abbreviation "NOS", the phrase "not elsewhere classified" (NEC), and the word "and" in titles. These need to be clearly understood by the coders.

1. Parentheses ( )

Parentheses are used in Volume 1 in four situations:

a) To *enclose additional or supplementary words*:

e.g. code I10-- *Hypertension* (arterial) (benign) (essential) (malignant) (primary) (systemic). It means that I10 is the code for *Hypertension* alone or when qualified by any of the words in parentheses. The presence or absence of terms enclosed in parentheses does not change the code number for that category.

b) To enclose the code to which an exclusion term refers. e.g. C00 *Malignant neoplasms of lip* excludes: skin of lip (C43.0, C44.0).

c) To enclose the three-character codes of categories included in a chapter or block, e.g. *Neoplasms* (C00-D48), *Malignant Neoplasms* (C00-C97).

d) To enclose the dagger code (✝) in an asterisk (*) category, e.g. G01* *Meningitis in Anthrax* (A22.8 ✝).

2. Square brackets [ ]

Square brackets are used:

a) For enclosing synonyms or alternative words, e.g.

A30 Leprosy [Hansen's disease]

B06 Rubella [German measles]

b) For referring to previous notes e.g. C00.8 *Overlapping lesion of lip* [See note 5 at the beginning of this chapter].

c) For referring to a previously stated set of four-character subdivisions common to a number of categories e.g. K27 *Peptic ulcer* [See before K25 for subdivisions].

3. Colon :

Terms followed by a colon (:) are not complete terms, but must have one of the understated modifiers to make them assignable to a given category:

> e.g. K36 OTHER APPENDICITIS
>> Appendicitis:
>> - chronic
>> - recurrent

The code number is not assigned to the term "Appendicitis", but to the term "chronic appendicitis" or "recurrent appendicitis". *Modifiers* (so called because they modify the meaning of the main term) appear after the colon sign. They are separated or preceded by bullets (.), which makes it easy to see which modifiers are essential.

4. Brace }

Braces are used to save space by reducing the amount of printed information in the tabular list of inclusions.

> e.g. J98.0 *Diseases of Bronchus, NEC*
>> Calcification
>> Stenosis $\Big\}$ of bronchus
>> Ulcer

Note that neither the words that precede it nor the words that are after it, are complete terms. Any of the term before the brace should be qualified by one or more of the terms that follow it, e.g.   calcification of bronchus

> stenosis of bronchus

> ulcer of bronchus

5.   "And" in titles

"And" in a title stands for and/or. For example, the category A18.0†, *Tuberculosis of bones and joints*, can cover:

Tuberculosis of bones
Tuberculosis of joints
Tuberculosis of bones *and* joints

6. Point dash

In some cases the 4th character of a sub-category code is replaced by a dash.

e.g. A06 *Amoebiasis*

> **excludes**: other protozoal intestinal diseases (A07.-)

A dash in the fourth position means that the category has been subdivided and you have to determine, by using the information given, which of those sub-categories is appropriate. In the above example, it means that the category A06 should only be used for *amoebiasis*. Any other protozoal intestinal disease belongs to category A07 and a number must replace the dash after the point (A07.-) specifying the protozoan causing the infection, e.g. A07.0 *Balantidiasis;* A07.1 *Giardiasis.*

7. NOS

NOS is an abbreviation for "NOT OTHERWISE SPECIFIED". It is equivalent to "unspecified" or "unqualified" and indicates where a disease belongs if it is not qualified. For example: Codes B15 to B19 list various forms of viral hepatitis (Chapter I). But if the physician has not specified which type of viral hepatitis (i.e. A, B, or C) the patient was suffering from, it is coded to B19.9 (Viral hepatitis NOS).

8. Not elsewhere classified (NEC)

This phrase when used in a 3-character category title indicates that certain specified variants of the listed conditions may appear in some other part of the classification and the coder must look for these before assigning this code. For example, the code R02 (*Gangrene, not elsewhere classified*) from chapter XVIII, may only be assigned if the disease cannot be coded more precisely from chapter IX (I70.2 *Atherosclerotic gangrene*), chapter IV (E10.5 *Diabetic gangrene*), or chapter I (A48.0 *Gas gangrene).*

Glossary descriptions

In addition to inclusion and exclusion terms, Chapter V (Mental and behavioural disorders) uses glossary descriptions to explain, in simple terms, the exact definition of morbid conditions listed there. This device is used because the terminology of mental disorders varies greatly, particularly between different countries, and the same name may be used to describe quite different conditions. The glossary is provided primarily to assist the diagnosticians. It is not intended for use by the coding staff.

Exercise 3.4

Mental retardation is a condition of arrested or incomplete development of the mind. It can be *mild, moderate, severe*, or *profound* as estimated by IQ tests. Locate code F73 in chapter V and,

1) Name the mental condition classified under it :
....
....

2) Write down the glossary definition of this condition:
....
....

Blocks

As stated earlier, the first grouping within ICD-10 occurs at the level of the chapter. Within each chapter, are found blocks of three-character categories grouped together. Blocks are shown in bold letters at the beginning of each chapter. A look at Chapter VIII (Diseases of the ear and mastoid process) in the list of Three-character categories will reveal four distinct blocks related to different disease conditions of the ear. Three of these include codes (H60-H83) for diseases associated with the three main structural parts of the ear (i.e. external, middle, and internal ear) while the fourth ("other disorders of ear") contains codes for various ill-defined conditions of the ear (H90-H95). This separation, into four parts, makes it easy for us to look at the total dimension of all ear diseases on a wider scale.

Categories

Within each block lie a number of categories related to a specific disease. For example, in the block "Diseases of external ear" (H60-H62), we find listed three main categories of disorders affecting the external ear, viz. *otitis externa* (H60), *other disorders of external ear* (H61), and *disorders of external ear in diseases classified elsewhere* (H62). These are called the *Three-character categories* as the codes they represent is made up of one letter of the alphabet, and two numbers, ranging from 00 to 99.

Subcategories

Most of the three-character categories are subdivided by means of a fourth, numeric character (0-9) after a decimal point, allowing up to ten Subcategories. The Four-character subcategories are used in whatever way is most appropriate -- identifying different sites or varieties if the three-character category is for a single disease [e.g. Paratyphoid fever 'A' (A01.1), Paratyphoid fever 'B' (A01.2), or Paratyphoid fever 'C' (A01.3)] or individual diseases if the Three-character category is for a group of conditions. For example, the Three-character category F60 (*specific personality disorders*) of chapter V (Mental and behavioural disorders) presents, in a subdivided form, and at the *fourth* character level, a number of specified disorders of personality, such as *Paranoid* (F60.0), *Schizoid* (F60.1), *Dissocial* (F60.2), *Aggressive* (F60.3), *Hysterical* (F60.4), among others.

Another example of subdivision at the Fourth-character level is B66 (*other fluke infections*) from Chapter I (Certain infectious and parasitic diseases) which provides a number of four-character codes for such individual parasitic conditions as *Opisthorchiasis* (B66.0), *Chlonorchiasis* (B66.1), *Dicrocoeliasis* (B66.2), *Fascioliasis* (B66.3) -- each caused by a specified parasitic worm, not classified elsewhere.

Whereas the fourth characters .0 – .7 are used for a specified site, variety or type of a disease condition, the character .8 is generally used for "other" conditions belonging to the Three-character category, and .9 is mostly used for an "unspecified" condition. For example, code K75.9 (*Hepatitis*) is allocated to unspecified hepatitis in case the patient records fail to mention if this hepatitis is acute, chronic, viral, bacterial, alcoholic, amoebic, or toxic.

Sub-categorization also exists at the *fifth* or subsequent character level, although it is not commonly encountered. An example of the *fifth-character* subdivision is to denote if a fracture is *closed* (0) or *open* (1). Thus "fracture of shaft of femur" may be coded as S72.30, if it is "closed" and S72.31, if specified as "open".

Illustrated summary

An example that would summarize the concept of chapter, block, category and sub category, and would make it amply clear, is taken from chapter X (Diseases of the respiratory system). There are ten main blocks into which all the respiratory conditions are grouped. The third block from the beginning is devoted to "acute lower respiratory infections" (other than pneumonia). You will notice that this block includes three categories -- J20 (*Acute bronchitis*), J21 (*Acute bronchiolitis*), and J22 (*Unspecified acute lower respiratory infections*). Let's consider the first category, J20 (*Acute bronchitis*), which is subdivided into ten subcategories ranging from J20.0 to J20.9. Each subcategory deals with a known specified cause of acute bronchitis. Usually, acute bronchitis is caused by one type of fungus (*Mycoplasma pneumoniae*), two types of bacteria (*Haemophilus influenzae and streptococcus*), and five types of viruses (*coxsackievirus, parainfluenza virus, syncytial virus, rhinovirus,* and *echovirus*). You will see that all eight of these main causative agents are represented by their individual subcategory and code (J20.0 to J20.7).

Acute bronchitis, however, is not caused by these eight agents only. There are "other", known etiological factors causing acute bronchitis, although less common. If the diagnosis indicates to one of these organisms, the name of which is *specified* on the patient records, and which is different from the already listed causative agents (J20.0 – J20.7), then this finds a place in a separate subcategory, J20.8, entitled "*Acute bronchitis due to other specified organisms*". However, if the patient records show no causative organisms and simply states the diagnosed condition as acute bronchitis, then it would belong to another subcategory at the very end, J20.9, appropriately entitled "*Acute bronchitis, unspecified*".

The following representation summarizes the structure of the main classification in a graphic form:

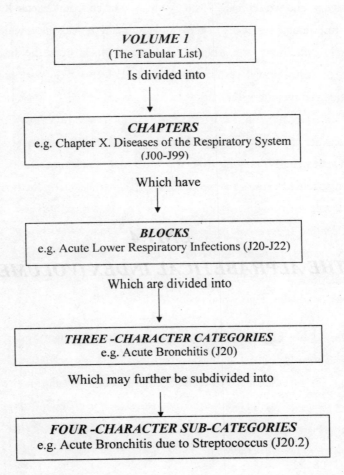

```
┌─────────────────────────────────────┐
│            VOLUME 1                  │
│         (The Tabular List)           │
└─────────────────────────────────────┘
            Is divided into
                  ↓

┌─────────────────────────────────────────┐
│               CHAPTERS                    │
│ e.g. Chapter X. Diseases of the Respiratory System │
│              (J00-J99)                    │
└─────────────────────────────────────────┘
            Which have
                  ↓

┌─────────────────────────────────────────┐
│                BLOCKS                     │
│ e.g. Acute Lower Respiratory Infections (J20-J22) │
└─────────────────────────────────────────┘
          Which are divided into
                  ↓

┌─────────────────────────────────────────┐
│      THREE -CHARACTER CATEGORIES         │
│        e.g. Acute Bronchitis (J20)       │
└─────────────────────────────────────────┘
      Which may further be subdivided into
                  ↓

┌─────────────────────────────────────────────┐
│      FOUR -CHARACTER SUB-CATEGORIES          │
│ e.g. Acute Bronchitis due to Streptococcus (J20.2) │
└─────────────────────────────────────────────┘
```

UNIT 4

THE ALPHABETICAL INDEX (VOLUME 3)

UNIT 4
THE ALPHABETICAL INDEX (VOLUME 3)

Introduction

Volume 3 of the International Classification of Diseases and Related Health Problem is an alphabetical index to the Tabular List of Volume 1 (Main Classification). It is an essential adjunct to the Tabular List and should be regarded as the primary coding tool. In fact, the two volumes must be used together, for the following reason:

The terms included in a category of the Tabular List (Volume 1) are not exhaustive; they serve as examples of the content of the category or as indicators of its extent and limits. The Index (Volume 3) on the other hand, is intended to include most of the diagnostic terms currently in use. Nevertheless, reference should always be made back to the Tabular List (Volume 1) and its notes, as well as to the guidelines provided in Volume 2, to ensure that the code given by the Index fits with the information provided by a particular patient record.

General arrangement of the Index

The Alphabetical Index consists of the three sections, as follows:
  I.   Alphabetical index to diseases and nature of injury
  II. External causes of injury
  III. Tables of drugs and chemicals

Section I

It is the index of diseases, syndromes, pathological conditions, injuries, signs, symptoms, problems and other reasons for contact with health services, i.e. the type of information that would be recorded by a physician. It includes all terms classifiable to categories A00-T98 and Z00-Z99 except drugs and other chemical substances leading to poisoning or other adverse effects (these are included in Section III). This section also includes a special table for **neoplasms**, classifying them according to sites and behaviour, i.e. benign, malignant, or unknown behaviour.

Section II

It is the index of all external causes of injury. The terms included here are not medical diagnoses but descriptions of the circumstances in which the violence occurred (e.g. fire, explosion, fall, assault, collision, drowning etc.). It includes all terms classifiable to V01-Y98, except drugs and chemicals.

Section III

It is the index of drugs and other chemical substances leading to poisoning or other adverse effects (referred to in Section I and II as the table of drugs and chemicals). For each substance the table gives the Chapter XIX code for poisoning (T36-T65) and the external cause (Chapter XX) codes for accidental poisoning by, and exposure to, noxious substances whether accidental or intentional (Y10-Y19). For drugs, medicaments and biological substances, it also gives the codes for these substances causing adverse effects in therapeutic use (Y40-Y59).

Exercise 4: In which volume of ICD-10 would you find the following? Put 1, 2, or 3 against your choice.

ITEM	VOLUME
a) List of 3-character categories	………..
b) History of ICD	………..
c) Table of drugs & chemicals	………..
d) Morphology of neoplasms.	………..
e) Statistical presentation	………..
f) Special tabulation lists	………
g) Rules and guidelines for using ICD-10	………

Structure of the Index

Each page of the Index (Section I & II) has two columns and located on the extreme left of each column is the **"lead term"** (usually a disease or pathological condition), which is printed in bold letters. Often the code for a particular condition is shown right against it. To illustrate the point, the first entry under the alphabet 'A' is "Aarskog's Syndrome". The ICD-10 code for this condition (Q87.1) is found right next to it. However, most lead terms have *qualifiers* or *modifiers* referring to the site (*Fracture of skull*), variety (*Viral hepatitis, Type A*), or cause of injury (*Burn by steam*) which are listed right under it, indented or separated by one, two, or more dashes depending upon the details of the diagnosed condition. For example, if the diagnosed condition is *Abnormal blood level of iron*, we can find it on the first page of the Index, listed under the letter 'A', and the lead term *Abnormal*. The next two components of the diagnosis, "*blood level of*" and "*iron*", can next be found separated by one and two dashes on the right, respectively, and enabling us to assign the most proper and precise code (R79.0) for this diagnostic condition.

Codes

The code numbers that follow the diagnostic terms refer to the *categories* and *subcategories* to which the terms should be classified. If the code has only three characters (e.g. B03, *Smallpox*) it can be assumed that the category has not been subdivided. In most cases where the category has been subdivided, the code number in the Index will give the fourth character (e.g. A20 *Plague*; A20.0 *Bubonic plague*). A dash in the fourth position (e.g. O03.- *Spontaneous abortion*) means that the category has been subdivided and that the fourth character can be found by referring to the Tabular list (003.4 *Incomplete abortion, without complication*, or 003.9 **Complete** *abortion, without* *complication*). If the dagger and asterisk system applies to the term, both codes are given (e.g. *Tuberculous meningitis*, A17.0✝ G01*).

Conventions used in the Index

There are certain conventions used throughout the Index, which you need to be aware of. These are explained below:

a) Parentheses ( )

Parentheses, or round brackets, are used to enclose words which may be present in a diagnosis but which are not essential. For example, look at the diagnostic statement "Diabetes" in Volume 3 (Index). You will notice that it has the following four terms in front of it, in parentheses: (*mellitus*), (*controlled*), (*familial*), and (*severe*) with the code E14.-. In means that E14.- is the code number for the word "Diabetes" alone or when qualified by the words in parentheses (i.e. *mellitus, controlled, familial, severe*). In other words, the word *mellitus*, or any one of the remaining three, may or may not appear in the diagnostic statement without affecting the way you code it.

b) NEC

The expression NEC ("Not Elsewhere Classified") in an Index term serves as a warning that other conditions, including the same term, may appear in other parts of the classification. An Index term followed by NEC should only be used after careful consideration and when it is quite clear that no information is available which would permit a more definite assignment, should the NEC term be used.

To illustrate the point, if you encounter the diagnostic statement "Food allergy" and if you look it up in the Index, you will see it coded as T78.1 (*Allergy, food* NEC T78.1). What it means is that you may assign this code *only* when the food source causing the allergic reaction is not specified. You must, at this point, look carefully in the patient records for other information. Perhaps this adverse reaction was caused due to some food borne bacteria, either specified or unspecified. In that case, choose a code from the category A05 (*Bacterial food borne intoxications*). The allergic reaction may also be due to other food sources such as *mushrooms* (T62.0), *berries* (T62.1), *seafood* (T61.0 – T61.9), or even food contaminants such as *mercury* (T56.1), *cyanides* (T65.0), or *mycotoxins* (T64). In brief, exhaust all possibilities before assigning T78.1 (*Allergy, food* NEC) as the code of choice.

c) Cross- references

Cross-references, such as "*see condition*", "*see*", and "*see also*", are used to avoid unnecessary duplication of entries in the Index. These useful terms are for your benefit when you cannot find a proper code for a particular diagnostic statement.

i) *See condition*: - You will not find anatomical sites (such as head, neck, leg, foot, liver, etc.) used as **lead terms** in the Index. For example, in the diagnosis *Fracture of neck*, if you look under *neck* (anatomical site) you will find *see condition*, in front of it. That means you should consult that part of the Index, which lists *fractures* of various anatomical sites. You will find *neck* listed there along with other anatomical sites. Read off the code against it (S12.9) and use it to code the condition.

ii) *See:* - Often you will not find the code for a condition that has been recorded by the doctor in an unconventional manner. For example, if a diagnosis reads "Allergic disorder, food", you look for it under "disorder, allergic" and find "*see* Allergy" written there. When you look under "Allergy" as directed, you will find "food" listed there and you should use it as the correct code (T78.1). Likewise, if you come across a diagnostic statement "Impaired hearing" and suppose you look for it under "Impaired" in the Index you will notice that mentioned against the qualifier "hearing", is a statement asking you to *see* Deafness. This indicates that the term "Impaired hearing" is to be coded in the same way as the term "Deafness". On looking up the latter term, you will find listed there various forms of deafness: *conductive, congenital, hysterical, ototoxic, syphilitic,* etc.

iii) *See also*: - Many conditions or disorders are known by more names than one. For example, "High blood pressure" is also known as "Hypertension". So, if you look for this you will easily find its code (I10). Note that you will find *See also* Hypertension, printed there. This tells you that "Hypertension" is an alternative term for "high blood pressure" and if you look under it ("Hypertension") you will find a long list of various kinds of high blood pressure caused by various conditions, giving you a greater choice in selecting the most appropriate code for your diagnosis. Similarly, if you come across "Lockjaw" as the diagnosed condition and find it in the Index it will give you one code for it (A35) and direct you to *see also* "Tetanus", where you will have the choice of choosing one from many, and hopefully, a more precise and appropriate code.

d) *Spelling*: -

American form of spelling is used for most terms in the Index. Users familiar with the British form should remember that the first letter of the vowel combinations "ae" (*anaemia*) and "oe" (*oedema*) and the "u" in words ending in "-our" (tumour) have been dropped, and the "re" (*goitre*) reversed to "er" in words ending thus. Thus the Index lists the above-mentioned terms as *anemia, edema, tumor,* and *goiter.*

e) Special signs

The following special signs will be found attached to certain code numbers or index terms:

    ✝ / * Used to designate the *etiology* code and *manifestation* code, respectively, for terms subject to dual classification (explained in greater detail in the next unit).

    # / ◊ Attached to certain terms in the list of sites under "Neoplasm" to refer the coder to Notes 2 and 3, respectively, at the start of that list (e.g. Neoplasm, *arm* NEC#; Neoplasm, *sternum* ◊; in the Index, Volume 3).

Categories with common characteristics

a) Asterisk categories

The following asterisk categories are not to be used alone. They must always be used in addition to a dagger code:

D63*, D77*, E35*, E90*, F00*, F02*, G01*, G02*, G05*, G07*, G13*, G22*, G26*, G32*, G46*, G53*, G55*, G59*, G63*, G73*, G94*, G99, H03*, H06*, H13*, H19*, H22*, H28*, H32*, H36*, H42*, H45*, H48*, H58*, H62*, H67*, H75*, H82*, H94*, I32*, I39*, I41*, I43*, I52*, I68*, I79*, I98*, J17*, J91*, J99*, K23*, K67*, K77*, K87*, K93*, L14*, L45*, L54*, L62*, L86*, L99*, M01*, M03*, M07*, M09*, M14*, M36*, M49*, M63*, M68*, M73*, M82*, M90*, N08*, N16*, N22*, N29*, N33*, N37*, N51*, N74*, N77*, P75*.

b) Categories limited to one sex

The following categories apply only to males:

B26.0, C60-C63, D07.4-D07.6, D17.6, D29.-, D40.-, E29.-, E89.5, F52.4, I86.1, L29.1, N40-N51, Q53-Q55, R86, S31.2-S31.3, Z12.5.

The following categories apply only to females:

A34, B37.3, C51-C58, C79.6, D06.-, D07.0-D07.3, D25-D28, D39.-, E28.-, E89.4, F52.5, F53.-, I86.3, L29.2, L70.5, M80.0-M80.1, M81.0-M81.1, M83.0, N70-N98, N99.2-N99.3, O00-O99, P54.6, Q50-Q52, R87, S31.4, S37.4-S37.6, T19.2-T19.3, T83.3, Y76.-, Z01.4, Z12.4, Z30.1, Z30.3, Z30.5, Z31.1, Z31.2, Z32-Z36, Z39.-, Z43.7, Z87.5, Z97.5.

c) Sequelae categories

The following categories are provided for sequelae of conditions that are no longer in an active phase:

B90-B94, E64.-, E68, G09, I69.-, O97, T90-T98, Y85-Y89.

d) Postprocedural disorders

The following categories are not to be used for underlying cause mortality coding.

E89.-, G97.-, H59.-, H95.-, I97.-, J95.-, K91.-, M96.-, N99.-.

UNIT 5
PRINCIPLES AND TECHNIQUES OF CODING

UNIT 5

PRINCIPLES AND TECHNIQUES OF CODING

Introduction

ICD allows us to allocate or translate the words used in a diagnosis to a specific code. This facilitates the grouping of diseases and conditions for statistical purposes. There has been a major change in the structure of the code in ICD-10 from that used in previous classifications when a number was used in the first position. Now, the ICD-10 codes start with a *letter* of the alphabet and are structured as follows:

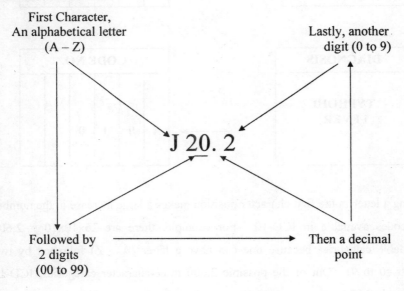

First Character,
An alphabetical letter
(A – Z)

Lastly, another
digit (0 to 9)

J 20. 2

Followed by
2 digits
(00 to 99)

Then a decimal
point

The first three characters, J20 in this example, refer to a *three-character category*," Acute Bronchitis ". The number following the decimal point—the fourth character – gives a code for a more specific subcategory of the disease or condition (J20.2 – "Acute Bronchitis due to Streptococcus"). This is referred to a *four- character subcategory.*

In some cases a three-character category is the code as there are no further qualifications. An example is: <u>B03</u> – "Smallpox". However, the vast majority of codes are four character codes. With this simple structure it is not difficult for you to translate:

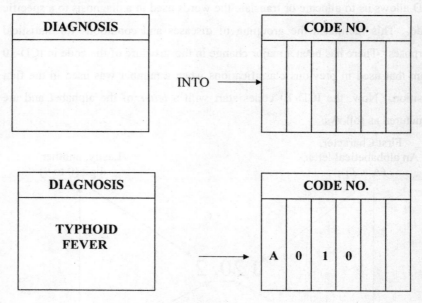

Using a letter in the first character position makes a large increase in the number of codes available in ICD-10. For example, there are 26x10x10 = 2,600 available categories because one can have a letter (A – Z) followed by two digits (0 to 9). Out of the possible 2,600 three-character categories, ICD-10 uses only 2,034.

Furthermore, since the majority of codes are four-character codes the potential number of codes is ten times greater than this (2600x10 = 26,000). In fact, about 10, 000 four-character codes are actually used in ICD-10.

How to code:

Entries in Section I and II of the Index are arranged in columns-- two on each page. In each column the term appearing on the extreme left is known as the "lead term". These terms are usually *nouns* indicating the name of a disease or condition. Before coding a diagnosis you must identify the disease or condition as a noun and use it as the lead term. If the diagnosis is expressed in the *adjective* form (i.e. "*Dislocated* shoulder"), convert it into the *noun* form (i.e. "*Dislocation of shoulder*") to obtain the lead term.

When using the Index to code eponymous diseases (diseases named after people, e.g. "*Down's* Syndrome", "*Alzheimer's* disease"), the lead term is the *name* and NOT the condition (i.e. syndrome, disease, etc.)

Exercise 5.1 Put the noun form of the italicized words on the left in the blank spaces on the right.

Adjective form	Noun (lead term)
1. A *sick* child	sickness
2. A *pregnant* lady	pregnancy
3. *Infected* tonsils	....
4. *Fractured* leg	....
5. *Contracted* muscle	....
6. *Defective* speech	....
7. *Transfused* blood	....
8. *Absent* ear	....
9. *Anemic* deficiency	....
10. *Complicated* delivery	....
11. *Diabetic* coma	....
12. *Allergic* medicine	....

After identifying the lead term you must refer to the appropriate section of the Alphabetical Index. If the diagnostic statement is a *disease* or *injury*, consult Section I of the Index. If the statement is the *external cause of an injury*, consult Section II. If the statement relates to *poisoning from a drug or chemical*, consult Section III.

Once you have identified the appropriate section and the lead term, you must now focus your attention on the *modifiers* or *qualifiers* in the diagnosis. In Section I, these modifiers refer to the variety, (such as "Hepatitis virus, *type A*"), site ("Fracture of *skull*"), or circumstance ("Exhaustion *due to cold*") that further describes the lead term. In Section III they indicate the various types of accident or occurrence (such as "burn by *hot water*", "*car* accident", etc.).

In the Index, these modifiers are indented (separated by one or more spaces to the right) under the lead term. There may be more than one modifier. Try to find as many of the modifiers as you can in the Index, which match exactly to the diagnosis that the doctor has recorded. Select that code which does full justice to all modifiers present in the diagnosis. You should then turn to Volume 1 and confirm that the selected code is the same at both places. Here is an example: - Suppose the doctor diagnoses the following condition:

Chronic viral hepatitis, type C

In this example, *Hepatitis is* the lead term, and the modifiers are *viral, chronic, type*, and '*C*'. You will find **Hepatitis**, the lead term, in Section I of the Index. The first modifier, *viral* is indented under it and marked by one dash (-); *chronic*, the second modifier, by two dashes (--); *type*, the third modifier, by three dashes (---); and lastly, '*C*', the fourth modifier, by four dashes (----). Select the code against the last modifier of the diagnosis (B18.2), ignoring all other entries in the list. Look at the graphic representation below to fully understand the selection process.

Hepatitis
- viral (acute) B19.9
- - chronic B18.9
- - - type
- - - - *C* B18.2

After noting down the selected code (B18.2), turn to Volume 1 (Tabular List) and find the page on which this code is listed and read the diagnostic statement appearing against.it for *confirmation*. Assign the code after ascertaining that all the words in the diagnostic expression have been accounted for.

Dual coding

By dual coding is meant having two codes for the same condition. There are certain situations that permit two ICD codes to be used to describe fully a person's condition. However, these additional codes are optional and would be used only in special tabulations.

a) The "Dagger and Asterisk" system

In this system there are two codes for diagnostic statements containing information about both an underlying generalized disease and a manifestation in a particular organ or site, which is a clinical problem in it, own right.

The primary code is for the *underlying disease* and is marked with a dagger (✝); an optional code for the *manifestation* is marked with an asterisk (*). For example, if the diagnostic statement is "Tuberculous meningitis" or "Diabetic retinopathy" and when you look for these in the Index you will find them coded as "Meningitis, tuberculous" A17.0✝G01*, and "Retinopathy, in diabetes" E14.3✝H36.0*, respectively. Here, the dagger (✝) stands for tuberculosis and diabetes, the two underlying diseases, and the asterisk (*) for meningitis and retinopathy, the two manifested conditions. In other words, the dagger code is used to identify the *disease, which caused the effect* and the asterisk code for identifying the *effect produced by the disease.*

While the dagger and asterisk system provides alternative classifications for the presentation of statistics, it is a principle of the ICD that the dagger code is the primary code and must always be used. Provision should be made for the asterisk code to be used *in addition* if the alternative method of presentation may also be required. For coding, *the asterisk code must never be used alone.*

The areas of the classification where the dagger and asterisk system operates are limited; there are 83 special asterisk categories throughout the classification, which are listed at the beginning of the relevant chapters.

Exercise 5.2 Find the primary and secondary codes for the diagnostic statement listed below and specify these against each statement.

CONDITION	PRIMARY CODE	SECONDARY CODE
1. Uremic pericarditis		
2. Gonococcal arthritis		
3. Mumps meningitis		
4. Tuberculous spondylitis		
5. Gouty iritis		

b) Other Optional dual coding systems

There are certain situations, other than in the dagger and asterisk system, identified by the note in the tabular list, "Use additional code, if desired..." that permit two ICD codes.

These are:

(i) For local infections, classifiable to the body system chapters,

codes from Chapter I may be added to identify the infecting organism, where this information does not appear in the title of the category (a block of categories, B95-B97, is provided for this purpose in Chapter I). A good example is the category G06 (Intracranial and intraspinal abscess and granuloma, Chapter VI, Volume1) that notifies the coder to "Use additional code (B95-B97), if desired, to identify the infectious agent".

(ii) For conditions classifiable to F00-F09 (organic, including symptomatic, mental disorders) in Chapter V, where a code from another chapter may be added to indicate the cause, i.e. the underlying disease, injury or other insult to brain. An example is category E00 (Congenital iodine-deficiency syndrome, Chapter IV) where a note tells the coder to "Use additional code F00-F79), if desired, to identify associated mental retardation".

(iii) For neoplasms, the morphology code from Volume 1, although not part of the main ICD, may be added to the Chapter II code to identify the morphological type of the tumour. An example is category D45 (Polycythaemia vera, Chapter II), where information exists about this neoplasm's morphological and behaviour code (M9950/1).

(iv) Where two codes can be used to describe an injury, poisoning or other adverse effect: a code from Chapter XIX, which describes the nature of the injury, and a code from Chapter XX, which describes the cause. For example, the diagnostic statement "Accidental poisoning by opium at home" can be given two codes, one from Chapter XIX (T40.0), and the other from Chapter XX (X42.0). Similarly, "Skull fracture from car accident, on street" may be expressed by two codes, S02.4 (Chapter XIX) and V49.9 (Chapter XX), extracted from Section II ("External Causes of Injury") of the Index.

Multiple diagnoses

The ICD provides certain categories where two conditions can be represented by a single code (e.g. Pneumoconiosis *with* tuberculosis, J65; Pleurisy *with* effusion, J90). The Alphabetical Index indicates where such combinations are provided for, under the indent "with", which appears immediately after the lead term.

Example ("Hernia with gangrene K46.1")

Hernia K46.9

- with

-- gangrene K46.1

Steps of coding

Coding from ICD-10 is a simple procedure if you know the principles of classification & coding as elaborated above. The ten basic steps of coding are listed below:

1. Carefully read the diagnostic statement as indicated by the doctor.

2. Refer to the appropriate section of the Alphabetical Index. For example:

   If it is a disease or injury: Consult Section I

   If it is the external cause of an injury: Consult Section II

   If it is related to a drug or chemical: Consult Section III

3. Identify the lead term. Convert it to a noun form if it is expressed in adjective form.

4. Look under the lead term for all qualifiers or modifiers.

5. Be guided by any inclusion or exclusion terms under the selected code, or under the chapter, block, or category heading. Also, pay attention to any note that appears under the lead term.

6. Follow carefully any cross references ("see", "see condition", and "see also") found in the references.

7. Take note of a category marked with the dagger and asterisk signs.

8. Find the fourth character in Volume 1 if the selected code is of three characters with a dash in the fourth position.

9. Refer to the Tabular List in Volume 1 to verify the suitability of the code number selected. Ensure that all the words in the diagnostic statement have been accounted for.

10. Assign the code.

UNIT 6
CHAPTER – CONTENTS ANALYSIS

CHAPTER I

Title: Certain Infectious & Parasitic Diseases

        Range of Codes: A00 – B99
        Number of Blocks: 21
        Available Categories: 200
        Allocated Categories: 171
        Asterisk Categories: None
        Chapter Type: Special Chapter

Introduction to the chapter

This is one of the largest chapters in ICD-10. It includes codes for the various types of infections caused by bacteria, viruses, fungi, protozoa, worms, and other parasites. It also has five well-defined codes (B20-24) for the HIV infection (AIDS), nonexistent in previous classifications.

Most common infectious and parasitic conditions coded from this chapter are: typhoid, T.B., cholera, smallpox, chickenpox, measles, plague, brucellosis, whooping cough, syphilis, gonorrhea, malaria, meningitis, mumps, hepatitis, helminthiasis, and HIV disease (AIDS).

Chapter-specific notes

Note the title carefully. The word "certain" means that some infectious and parasitic conditions (such as influenza, perinatal infections, etc.) are classified elsewhere. Look at the "Excludes" list at the beginning of the chapter for more of these conditions. Also, read carefully the beginning "note" of category A09 before classifying diarrhea and gastroenteritis.

Exercise 6.1 Circle either T (True) or F (False) after carefully studying the Three-character and Four-character lists of Chapter I.

1. Salmonella infections are intestinal infections.   T   F

2. Gonococcal infections have a predominantly sexual
   mode of transfer.   T   F

3. Typhus fever is an example of Rickettsiosis.   T   F

4. Filariasis is a bacterial disease.   T   F

5. HIV Disease is a protozoan disease.   T   F

6. *Varicella* is another name for chickenpox.   T   F

7. Diarrhoea of all types can be coded from this chapter.   T   F

8. Rabies is a viral infection of the Central Nervous
   System.   T   F

CODING EXERCISE – CHAPTER I

I. Using Volume 3 (Index) of ICD-10, provide appropriate codes for the following diagnostic statements:

No.	Diagnostic statements	ICD-10 code
1	Paratyphoid fever, C	
2	Congenital Syphilis	
3	Falciparum malaria with cerebral complications	
4	Ascariasis with intestinal complications	
5	Salmonella enteritis	
6	Tuberculosis of lung	
7	Candidiasis of nails	
8	Sequelae of genitourinary tuberculosis	
9	Pediculosis capitis	
10	Streptococcal infection	
11	Taenia saginata infection	
12	Tetatnus neonatorum	
13	Tonsillar diphtheria	
14	Cholera	
15	Acute amebic dysentery	
16	Chronic viral hepatitis, type C	
17	Brucellosis due to Brucella canis	
18	Tuberculoid leprosy	
19	German measles	
20	Viral conjunctivitis	

II. Using Volume 1 (Four-Character Categories, Tabular List), provide *complete* diagnostic statements for the following codes:

No.	ICD-10 code	Diagnostic statement
1	A40.0	
2	B05.4	
3	A36.9	
4	B23.0	
5	A18.0†	

CHAPTER II

Title: Neoplasms

> Range of Codes: C00 – D48
> Number of Blocks: 4
> Available Categories: 149
> Allocated Categories: 136
> Asterisk Categories: None
> Chapter Type: Special Chapter

Introduction to the chapter

This chapter provides codes for all diagnostic entries specified as neoplasm, cancer, tumor, mass, growth, lump, etc. All neoplasms in this chapter are classified by site or location (e.g. brain, skin, bone) and divided into four major blocks covering malignant, benign, in situ, and neoplasms of uncertain or unknown behaviour. Of these, the block including the malignant neoplasms is the largest, divided into 15 sub-blocks and 88 categories.

Chapter-specific notes

1. In addition to *site*, neoplasms are also classified according to the arrangement of cells or tissues as seen under the microscope (in other words, according to the MORPHOLOGY of the neoplasms). Some common examples of morphological terms are adenoma, papilloma, melanoma, carcinoma, lipoma, myeloma, sarcoma, fibroma, etc. You will *not* find morphological codes in this chapter. There is a separate section for this at the end of Volume 1.

2. In coding neoplasms from this chapter, ensure that you use the special table for this purpose in Volume 3 (Index), under the lead terms **Neoplasm, Neoplastic**.

3. The table shows five columns against each neoplasmic site to let you choose the appropriate code depending upon its behaviour (i.e. malignant, benign, in situ, etc.).

4. Be guided by a set of eight notes at the beginning of the chapter before assigning a code from this chapter.

Exercise 6.2

Identify, from the list on the left, which letter (S, M, or B) corresponds to the terms on the right:

	1. Benign ......
	2. Skin ......
Site (S)	3. Lipoma ......
	4. Malignant ......
Morphology (M)	5. Bone ......
	6. Sarcoma ......
Behavior (B)	7. in situ ......
	8. Liver ......
	9. Melanoma ......
	10. Adenoma ......

CODING EXERCISE – CHAPTER II

I. Using Volume 3 (Index) of ICD-10, provide appropriate codes for the following diagnostic statements:

No.	Diagnostic statements	ICD-10 code
1	Brain tumour, benign	
2	Skin cancer of uncertain behavior	
3	Bronchial carcinoma, secondary	
4	Malignant mass of face, primary	
5	Carcinoma of posterior stomach wall, secondary	
6	In situ neoplasm of internal auditory canal	
7	Malignant lump of inner ear, primary	
8	Lung tumour of unknown behavior	
9	Benign neoplasm of cervix canal	
10	Neoplasm of lingual tonsil, benign	
11	Malignant neoplasm of nasal cavity, primary	
12	Uterine cancer of uncertain behavior	
13	In situ neoplasm of the skin of leg	
14	Benign neoplasm of ventral surface of tongue	
15	Malignant lump of vulva, secondary	
16	Malignant mass of chin, primary	
17	Neoplasm of upper gum, benign	
18	Breast tumor of uncertain behavior	
19	Benign neoplasm of bladder neck	
20	Carcinoma of wrist bone, secondary	

II. Using Volume 1 (Four-Character Categories, Tabular List), provide *complete* diagnostic statements for the following codes:

No.	ICD-10 code	Diagnostic statement
1	D48.6	
2	C25.9	
3	D10.2	
4	D06.0	
5	D30.3	

CHAPTER III

Title: Diseases of the blood & blood forming organs and certain disorders involving the immune mechanism

> Range of Codes: D50-D89
> Number of Blocks: 6
> Available Categories: 40
> Allocated Categories: 34
> Asterisk Categories: 2
> Chapter Type: Special chapter

Introduction to the Chapter

This is the shortest chapter within ICD-10. It has been split into 6 blocks, with the first three covering anemias (nutritional, hemolytic, aplastic), the fourth dealing with coagulation defects, the fifth with certain other diseases of blood-forming organs, and the sixth with certain disorders involving the immune mechanism.

Chapter-specific notes

Be cautious in not making an attempt to code HIV disease (AIDS) from this chapter just because the title indicates that the chapter contains certain disorders involving the immune mechanism. This fact is emphasized in the exclusion list at the beginning of the chapter.

Exercise 6.3

I. One immunity disorder is excluded from this chapter because it appears in chapter I. Name it and specify the codes assigned to it.

a) Name of the disorder: ....

b) Codes assigned: ....

II. From the list of conditions in column I choose the ones that belong to respective anaemia groups in column II and place its number(s) in the blank space on extreme right.

COLUMN I	COLUMN II	NO.
1. Thalassaemia	Nutritional Anaemias	......
2. Vitamin B12 Deficiency		
3. Erythroblastopenia	Haemoloytic Anaemias	......
4. Sickle-cell disorders		
5. Folate deficiency anaemia	Aplastic Anaemias	......
6. Acute posthemorrhagic anaemia		

CODING EXERCISE – CHAPTER III

I. Using Volume 3 (Index) of ICD-10, provide appropriate codes for the following diagnostic statements:

No.	Diagnostic statements	ICD-10 code
1	Hemophilia, type C	
2	Neutropenic splenomegaly	
3	Hereditary eosinophilia	
4	Drug induced nonautoimmune hemolytic anemia	
5	Von Willebrand disease	
6	Christmas disease	
7	Idiopathic thrombocytopenic purpura	
8	Constitutional aplastic anemia	
9	Chronic red cell aplasia	
10	Paroxysmal nocturnal hemoglobinuria	
11	Deficiency of factor XII	
12	Sickle-cell trait	
13	Iron deficiency anemia	
14	Vascular pseudohemophilia	
15	Agranulocytosis	
16	Abscess of spleen	
17	Gray platelet syndrome	
18	Congenital dysphagocytosis	
19	Sarcoidosis of lymph nodes and lung	
20	Vitamin B12 deficiency anemia	

II. Using Volume 1 (Four-character categories, Tabular List, provide *complete* diagnostic statements for the following codes:

No.	ICD-10 code	Diagnostic statement
1	D56.0	
2	D72.1	
3	D57.0	
4	D73.5	
5	D50.9	

CHAPTER IV

Title: Endocrine, Nutritional and Metabolic Diseases
Range of Codes: E00-E90
Number of Blocks: 8
Available Categories: 91
Allocated Categories: 73
Asterisk Categories: 2
Chapter Type: Special Chapter

Introduction to the chapter: This chapter includes the following:-

1. Disorders of the Endocrine glands (hypo-or hyper secretion of the thyroid, pituitary, adrenal, gonads, thymus, and pancreas glands). Examples: goiter, Cushing's disease, acromegaly, diabetes mellitus, etc. Codes: E00-E35.

2. **Nutritional Disorders** (Disorders due to malnutrition and deficiencies of proteins, vitamins or minerals). Examples: marasmus, kwashiorkor, deficiency of Vitamin A, B, C, D, E, & K, obesity. Codes E40-E68.

3. **Metabolic Disorders** (Disorders of physical and chemical processes by which energy derived from food and oxygen is made available to body tissues (Examples: cystic fibrosis, amyloidosis, acidosis, alkalosis, lactose intolerance, dehydration, etc.) Codes: E70-E90.

Chapter-specific notes

1. You may code dehydration due to fluid depletion from this chapter but apply care and classify dehydration of the newborn elsewhere (code P74.1)

2. The five codes assigned to diabetes mellitus (E10-E14) are of three characters only and the fourth character (.0-.9) *must be supplied* using the list before these codes, as suggested by a note to this effect.

3. Be guided by glossary description of terms related to malnutrition disorders (E40-E43, E44.0 and E44.1).

Exercise 6.4   Circle what you think are either True (T) or False (F) statements.

1. Cystic fibrosis is a nutritional disorder.   T   F

2. Obesity is a metabolic disorder.   T   F

3. Goitre is an endocrine disorder.   T   F

4. One example of nutritional disorders is lactose
   intolerance.   T   F

5. Kwashiorkor is an endocrine disorder.   T   F

6. Complications of pregnancy, childbirth, and
   puerparium can be coded from this chapter.   T   F

CODING EXERCISE – CHAPTER IV

I. Using Volume 1 (Tabular List) and Volume 3 (Index) of the ICD-10,
Provide appropriate codes for the following diagnostic statements:

No.	Diagnostic statements	ICD-10 code
1	Insulin-dependent diabetes mellitus, with coma	
2	Drug-induced hypoglycemia with coma (nondiabetic)	
3	Drug-induced Cushing's syndrome	
4	Pituitary gigantism	
5	Marasmic kwashiorkor	
6	Third degree malnutrition	
7	Vitamin A deficiency with conjunctival xerosis	
8	Obesity due to excess calories	
9	Classical phenylketonuria	
10	Non-insulin-dependent diabetes mellitus with ketoacidosis	
11	Hypercholesterolemia with Hyperglyceridemia	
12	Cystic fibrosis with intestinal manifestations	
13	Iron deficiency	
14	Hyperthyroidism with diffuse goiter	
15	Polycystic ovarian syndrome	
16	Non-insulin-dependent diabetes with unspecified complications	
17	Idiopathic hypoparathyroidism	
18	Thiamine deficiency with beriberi	
19	Lactose intolerance	
20	Insulin-dependent diabetes mellitus, with renal complications	

II. Using Volume 1 (Four-Character Categories, Tabular List), provide *complete* diagnostic statements for the following codes:

No.	ICD-10 code	Diagnostic statement
1	E84.1	
2	E87.4	
3	E10.4	
4	E50.5	
5	E11.9	

CHAPTER V

Title: Mental & Behavioural Disorders

Range of Codes: F00-F99
Number of Blocks: 11
Available Categories: 100
Allocated Categories: 78
Asterisk Categories: 2
Chapter Type: Special Chapter

Introduction to the chapter

This chapter covers a range of disorders in which there is some kind of abnormal functioning of the mind. You will notice the presence of "glossary descriptions" (definitions to explain terms) in this chapter. These are provided to guide the doctors (psychiatrists) when choosing the correct diagnostic terms as in the field of mental disorders there is much more variation than usual between doctors as to the name they give to the various problems.. The following is a list of most frequently encountered disorders from this chapter: schizophrenia, neuroses, psychoses, phobias, dementia, alcoholism, personality disorders, drug dependence, depression, eating disorders, delirium, hallucination, and mental retardation.

Chapter-specific notes

1. The definitions of the categories and sub-categories (Glossary Descriptions) in this chapter are provided to assist the doctors in establishing diagnostic labels. You, the coder, can read these glossaries but you should not use them, as your main task is to code the terms used by the doctor, not to interpret them.

There are two set of categories where you are advised to use a fourth-character, ranging from .0 to .9. The first one (F10-F19) specifies the clinical state in psychoactive substance use, and the other (F70-79) identifies the extent of impairment of behaviour in mental retardation.

Exercise 6.5

Circle either True (T) or False (F) where appropriate.

1. Behavioural disorders cannot be coded from
   this chapter.   T   F

2. Glossary pertains to the definition of terms.   T   F

3. Glossaries can be used by *coders* in finding
   appropriate codes.   T   F

4. Tobacco abuse can be coded from this chapter.   T   F

5. There is no code for mental retardation in this
   chapter.   T   F

CODING EXERCISE – CHAPTER V

I. Using Volume 3 (Index) of the ICD-10, provide appropriate codes for the following diagnostic statements:

No.	Diagnostic statements	ICD-10 code
1	Dementia of old age	
2	Anxiety disorder due to alcohol	
3	Obsessional rituals	
4	Dissociative sensory loss	
5	Undifferentiated somatoform disorder	
6	Atypical bulimia nervosa	
7	Hopochondrical disorder	
8	Anorexia nervosa	
9	Depersonalization – derealization syndrome	
10	Acute stress reaction	
11	Hyperkinetic disorder	
12	Excessive thumb-sucking in childhood	
13	Nocturnal psychogenic enuresis	
14	Developmental learning disorder	
15	Catatonic schizophrenia	
16	Delirium due to alcohol withdrawal	
17	Separation anxiety disorder of childhood	
18	Organic hallucinosis	
19	Bipolar affective disorder, unspecified	
20	Sibling rivalry disorder	

II. Using Volume I (Four-Character Categories, Tabular List), provide *complete* diagnostic statements for the following codes:

No.	ICD-10 code	Diagnostic statement
1	F30.2	
2	F50.2	
3	F72.0	
4	F20.0	
5	F41.1	

CHAPTER VI

Title: Disorders of the Nervous System

Range of Codes: G00-G99
Number of Blocks: 11
Available Categories: 100
Allocated Codes: 67
Asterisk Categories: 16
Chapter Type: Body System Chapter

Introduction to the chapter

This chapter covers diseases of the:

1. Central Nervous System (brain & spinal cord)
2. Peripheral Nervous System (nerve network)

There are three terms, which you will find repeatedly used, in various forms, in this chapter. These are, *encephalon* (tissues of the brain), *myelo* (tissues of spinal cord), and *meninges* (membranes covering the brain and spinal cord). Inflammation of these nerve tissues leads to specific diseases that you will find listed in this chapter. Some frequently encountered examples of disorders from this chapter are: epilepsy, migraine, sleep disorders, meningitis, encephalitis, Parkinson's disease, Alzheimer's disease, cerebral palsy, hemiplegia & paraplegia, hydrocephalus, and multiple sclerosis.

Chapter-specific notes

1. As most diseases of this chapter are infectious they are primarily assigned a code in Chapter I, which deals exclusively with infectious diseases. This explains why many of the diseases included in this chapter are given asterisk codes. When you come across any of these, either write both codes, or if only one code is required, choose the dagger code from Chapter I.

2. Pay attention to the note under the category G09 (sequelae of inflammatory diseases of central nervous system). The"sequelae" include conditions specified as such or as late effects, or those present one year or more after onset of the causal condition.

3. Categories G81 (Hemiplegia), G82 (Paraplegia) and G83 (Other paralytic syndromes) should be used only when the listed conditions are reported without further specification, or are stated to be old or longstanding but of unspecified cause.

Exercise 6.6

Fill in the blank spaces:

1. Inflammation of................................. leads to meningitis.

2. Myelitis refers to the .... of the spinal cord.

3. .... refers to the inflammation of brain tissue.

4. Most dagger codes referred to in this chapter can be found in chapter
   ....

5. Central nervous system includes brain and ....

CODING EXERCISE – CHAPTER VI

I. Using Volume 3 (Index) of the ICD-10, provide appropriate codes
for the following diagnostic statement:

No.	Diagnostic statements	ICD-10 code
1	Migraine without aura	
2	Parkinson's disease	
3	Circumscribed brain atrophy	
4	Alzheimer's disease, late onset	
5	Drug-induced chorea	
6	Multiple sclerosis	
7	Epilepsy	
8	Cluster headache syndrome	
9	Sleep disorder	
10	Carpal tunnel syndrome	
11	Idiopathic progressive neuropathy	
12	Myasthenia gravis	
13	Muscular dystrophy	
14	Flaccid paraplegia	
15	Spastic hemiplegia	
16	Ataxic cerebral palsy	
17	Compression of brain	
18	Obstructive hydrocephalus	
19	Alcoholic myopathy	
20	Eaton-Lambert syndrome	

II. Using Volume 1 (Four-Character Categories, Tabular List), provide *complete* diagnostic statements for the following codes:

No.	ICD-10 code	Diagnostic statement
1	G80.0	
2	G00.2	
3	G20	
4	G30	
5	G40.3	

CHAPTER VII

Title: Diseases of the Eye & Adnexa

> Range of Codes: H00-H59
> Number of Blocks: 11
> Available Categories: 60
> Allocated Categories: 47
> Asterisk Categories: 12
> Chapter Type: Body System Chapter

Introduction to the chapter

This chapter provides codes for the diseases of the eye and adnexa. The word *adnexa* means, "associated parts" and here includes such structures as eyelids, tear glands, optic nerve, orbit, eye muscles, etc. The blocks in this chapter are mainly arranged in anatomical sequence. This arrangement is designed to provide a logical layout to the chapter and to help coders when they are looking up specific diseases and conditions. Some frequently occurring examples from this chapter are: conjunctivitis, keratitis, iritis, corneal opacity, cataract, glaucoma, strabismus, visual disturbances, and blindness.

Chapter-specific notes

The code H54 (Blindness and low vision) should *not* be used as the main condition if the cause for blindness & low vision is given, unless the episode of care was mainly for the blindness itself. Also, the table classifying the severity of visual impairment is primarily for use by doctors when writing a diagnosis, and *not* for the coders.

Exercise 6.7

Circle either True (T) or False (F):

1. Tear glands are not part of adnexa.   T   F

2. There are no asterisk categories in this chapter.   T   F

3. Strabismus is an eye disorder.   T   F

4. Code H54 should always be used as the main condition when coding blindness or low vision.   T   F

5. Table classifying the severity of visual impairment is mainly for the use of coders.   T   F

CODING EXERCISE – CHAPTER VII

I. Using Volume 3 (Index) of the ICD-10, provide appropriate codes for the following diagnostic statement:

No.	Diagnostic statements	ICD-10 code
1	Vertical strabismus	
2	Sudden visual loss	
3	Hypermetropia	
4	Hereditary choroidal dystrophy	
5	Hordeolum	
6	Chalazion	
7	Blepharitis	
8	Deformity of orbit	
9	Pterygium	
10	Corneal ulcer	
11	Keratitis	
12	Traumatic cataract	
13	Low-tension glaucoma	
14	Traction detachment of retina	
15	Vitreous hemorrhage	
16	Double vision	
17	Astigmatism	
18	Senile nuclear cataract	
19	Blindness, one eye	
20	Lens-induced iridocyclitis	

II. Using Volume 1 (Four-Character Categories, Tabular List), provide *complete* diagnostic statements for the following codes:

No.	ICD-10 code	Diagnostic statement
1	H54.0	
2	H10.1	
3	H26.3	
4	H40.1	
5	H49.9	

CHAPTER VIII

Title: Diseases of the Ear and Mastoid Process

Range of Codes: H60-H95
Number of Blocks: 4
Available Categories: 36
Allocated Categories: 24
Asterisk Categories: 5
Chapter Type: Body System Chapter

Introduction to the chapter

This chapter provides codes for important diseases of the ear and mastoid process. The mastoid process is the projecting portion of the temporal bone behind the ear. It contains numerous air passages, which can become infected causing mastoiditis. There is a simple structure to this chapter. The main blocks are divided on an anatomical basis into diseases of the:

a) External ear
b) Middle ear and mastoid
c) Inner ear
d) Other disorders of ear

The last group (H90-H95) covers disorders, which cannot be precisely classified in the previous blocks. The most frequently encountered conditions from this chapter are: otitis media, impacted cerumen (ear wax), Eustachian salpingitis, mastoiditis, vertigo, otosclerosis, tinnitus, otalgia, otorrhea, and hearing loss.

Chapter-specific notes

Codes H90 and H91 (Hearing loss) should not be used as the preferred codes for the main condition if the exact cause of hearing loss is recorded, unless the episode of care was mainly for the hearing loss itself.

Exercise 6.8

Circle either T (True) or F (False)

1. The term "impacted cerumen" means wax in
   the ear.   T   F
2. Mastoid process is a part of the temporal bone.   T   F
3. Otalgia cannot be coded from this chapter.   T   F
4. Otitis media refers to the infected air passages
   of the mastoid process.   T   F
5. This is a body system chapter.   T   F

CODING EXERCISE – CHAPTER VIII

I. Using Volume 3 (Index) of the ICD-10, provide appropriate codes
for the following diagnostic statement:

No.	Diagnostic statements	ICD-10 code
1	Tinnitus	
2	Otorrhea	
3	Conductive hearing loss, bilateral	
4	Disorder of eighth cranial nerve	
5	Sudden (idiopathic) deafness	
6	Polyp of middle ear	
7	Meniere's disease	
8	Acoustic trauma	
9	Cochlear otosclerosis	
10	Lermoyez' syndrome	
11	Eustachian salpingitis	
12	Acute mastoiditis	
13	Chronic myringitis	
14	Presbycusis	
15	Abscess of external ear	
16	Chronic mucoid otitis media	
17	Labyrinthine dysfunction	
18	Sensorineural hearing loss, bilateral	
19	Obstruction of eustachian tube	
20	Perichondritis of external ear	

II. Using Volume 1 (Four-Character Categories, Tabular List), provide *complete* diagnostic statements for the following codes:

No.	ICD-10 code	Diagnostic statement
1	H66.0	
2	H61.2	
3	H72.0	
4	H81.1	
5	H91.9	

CHAPTER IX

Title: Diseases of the Circulatory System

Range of Codes: I00-I99
Number of Blocks: 10
Available Categories: 100
Allocated Categories: 77
Asterisk Categories: 8
Chapter Type: Body System Chapter

Introduction to the chapter

Chapter IX covers diseases of the circulatory system, dealing with diseases of those parts involved with the circulation of blood and lymph. These are: heart, arteries, veins, and lymphatic system. It does not include diseases of the blood itself, which are covered in Chapter III. You may wonder why rheumatic fever is included in this chapter. Well rheumatic fever is a complication following a streptococcal infection such as severe sore throat or scarlet fever, which may result in serious heart damage. Therefore it is classified in this chapter.

Most common examples from this chapter are:
Rheumatic heart disease, hypertension & hypotension, pulmonary embolism, heart failure, heart valve disease, atherosclerosis, aneurism, cerebral thrombosis (stroke), haemorrhoids, varicose veins, etc.

Chapter-specific notes

The time elapsing between onset and care, or onset and death is important when classifying categories I21-I25 (Ischaemic heart diseases). Take note that a condition must have existed up to a period of 28 days (4 weeks) in order to be classified as *acute* (codes I21-I24).

Exercise 6.9

Circle either T (True) or F (False)

1. There are 100 allocated categories in this chapter.   T   F
2. This chapter does not include diseases of the blood
   itself.   T   F
3. Scarlet fever can be coded from this chapter.   T   F
4. Angina pectoris is an example of ischaemic heart
   disease.   T   F
5. Chronic ischaemic heart disease is considered to be
   more longstanding than 28 days (4 weeks).   T   F

CODING EXERCISE – CHAPTER IX

I. Using Volume 3 (Index) of the ICD-10, provide appropriate codes
for the following diagnostic statement:

No.	Diagnostic statements	ICD-10 code
1	Atherosclerosis of aorta	
2	Raynaud's syndrome	
3	Rupture of artery	
4	Phlebitis of femoral vein	
5	External thrombosed hemorrhoids	
6	Varicose veins of lower extremities with ulcer	
7	Esophageal varices with bleeding	
8	Hypotension due to drugs	
9	Cardiac arrest	
10	Postcardiotomy syndrome	
11	Necrosis of artery	
12	Atherosclerosis of renal artery	
13	Moyamoya disease	
14	Cerebral infarction	
15	Cardiac septal defect, acquired	
16	Sick sinus syndrome	
17	Ventricular fibrillation	
18	Occlusion of vertebral artery	
19	Supraventricular tachycardia	
20	Sudden cardiac death	

II. Using Volume 1 (Four-Character Categories, Tabular List), provide *complete* diagnostic statements for the following codes:

No.	ICD-10 code	Diagnostic statement
1	I11	
2	I20.0	
3	I50.1	
4	I72.0	
5	I05.9	

CHAPTER X

Title: Disorders of the Respiratory System

Range of Codes: J00-J99
Number of Blocks: 10
Available Categories: 100
Allocated Categories: 63
Asterisk Categories: 3
Chapter Type: Body System Chapter

Introduction to the chapter

This chapter covers diseases affecting the respiratory system. The classification follows an anatomical progression starting with the upper respiratory tract (nose, nasal sinuses, tonsils, larynx, vocal cords) and proceeding to the lower respiratory tract (bronchus, bronchioles, lung, interstitium, and pleura). The main diseases affecting the U.R.T. (upper respiratory tract) are the consequences of infections or allergies. Lung diseases are mainly the result of various reactions of the lungs to factors such as infections and inhaled pollutants.

Some commonly occurring diagnoses from this chapter are: common cold, sinusitis, tonsillitis, laryngitis, tracheitis, influenza, pneumonia, bronchitis, asthma, emphysema, pneumoconioses, pulmonary edema, pneumothorax, abscess of lung & mediastinum, pyothorax, etc.

Chapter-specific notes

1. Be careful in coding *Pneumonia* from this chapter. You may encounter such diagnoses as congenital pneumonia; interstitial pneumonia; pneumonia associated with measles, chickenpox, German measles, or rheumatic fever; and pneumonia due to typhoid fever, gonorrhea, or

whooping cough. In such cases (mostly J17 sub-categories) select the appropriate dagger code as indicated in the parentheses.

2. When a respiratory condition is described as occurring in more than one site and is not specifically indexed, it should be classified to the lower anatomic site.

3. Bronchitis not specified as acute or chronic in those less than 15 years of age can be assumed to be of acute nature and should be classified to J20.

Exercise 6.10

Specify, by putting 'U' against the following organs, if they belong to the upper respiratory tract or by 'L' if to the lower respiratory tract.

ORGANS	RESPIRATORY TRACT
1. Nasal sinuses	....
2. Lung	....
3. Nose	....
4. Bronchus	....
5. Tonsils	....
6. Bronchioles	....
7. Vocal cords	....
8. Larynx	....
9. Pleura	....
10. Interstitium	....

CODING EXERCISE – CHAPTER X

I. Using Volume 3 (Index) of the ICD-10, provide appropriate codes
for the following diagnostic statement:

No.	Diagnostic statements	ICD-10 code
1	Common cold	
2	Acute respiratory failure	
3	Streptococcal pharyngitis	
4	Acute maxillary sinusitis	
5	Fibrothorax	
6	Nonallergic asthma	
7	Pneumoconiosis due to talc dust	
8	Viral pneumonia with influenza	
9	Chronic pneumothorax	
10	Chronic obstructive pulmonary disease	
11	MacLeod's syndrome	
12	Simple chronic bronchitis	
13	Chronic laryngitis	
14	Chronic disease of tonsils and adenoids	
15	Polyp of nasal cavity	
16	Allergic rhinitis due to pollen	
17	Pneumonia due to pseudomonas	
18	Acute bronchiolitis	
19	Stenosis of larynx	
20	Centrilobular emphysema	

II. Using Volume 1 (Four-Character Categories, Tabular List), provide
complete diagnostic statements for the following codes:

No.	ICD-10 code	Diagnostic statement
1	J20.6	
2	J60	
3	J34.2	
4	J85.1	
5	J03.0	

CHAPTER XI

Title: Diseases of the Digestive System

> Range of Codes: K00-K93
> Number of Blocks: 10
> Available Categories: 94
> Allocated Categories: 71
> Asterisk Categories: 5
> Chapter Type: Body System Chapter

Introduction to the chapter

This chapter covers disorders of the digestive system. The first six blocks of the chapter deal with the components of the G.I (gastrointestinal) tract in a sequential order i.e. from mouth to anus. The following three blocks deal with the disorders of peritoneum, liver, and pancreas. The last block covers intestinal malabsorption and other residual disorders of the digestive system.

Some common examples of this chapter are:

Dental disorders, gastric & duodenal ulcers, gastritis and enteritis, dyspepsia, appendicitis, hernias, colitis, anal fissures and fistulas, peritonitis, cirrhosis & hepatitis, cholelithiasis, cholecyctitis, pancreatitis, etc.

Chapter-specific notes

1. Pay special attention to the note preceding code K25 concerning 4th character sub-divisions of the various ulcers of the upper G.I. tract as you will have to assign these codes yourself in accordance with the diagnosis giving you the behavior & type of the ulcer.

2. Classify "Hernia with gangrene _and_ obstruction" as "Hernia with gangrene".

Exercise 6.11

Circle either T (True) or F (False):

1. This chapter is a special chapter.   T   F
2. The last block of this chapter covers the various intestinal malabsorption disorders.   T   F
3. There are no asterisk categories in this chapter.   T   F
4. Diabetes can be coded from this chapter.   T   F
5. Code K27.1 refers to acute peptic ulcer with perforation.   T   F

CODING EXERCISE – CHAPTER XI

I. Using Volume 3 (Index) of the ICD-10, provide appropriate codes for the following diagnostic statement:

No.	Diagnostic statements	ICD-10 code
1	Toxic liver disease with acute hepatitis	
2	Cyst of pancreas	
3	Gastrointestinal hemorrhage	
4	Celiac disease	
5	Hernia with gangrene and obstruction .	
6	Postoperative intestinal obstruction	
7	Acute pancreatitis	
8	Acute gastric ulcer with perforation	
9	Alcoholic gastritis	
10	Atrophy of tongue papillae	
11	Vesicular stomatitis	
12	Chronic gingivitis	
13	Abrasion of teeth	
14	Teething syndrome	
15	Radicular cyst	
16	Gingival recession	
17	Acute appendicitis with generalized peritonitis	
18	Crohn's disease of large intestine	
19	Anorectal fistula	
20	Functional diarrhea	

II. Using Volume 1 (Four-Character Categories, Tabular List), provide *complete* diagnostic statements for the following codes:

No.	ICD-10 code	Diagnostic statement
1	K26.0	
2	K35.1	
3	K41.1	
4	K28.5	
5	K72.1	

CHAPTER XII

Title: Disorders of the Skin and Subcutaneous Tissue

Range of Codes: L00-L99
Number of Blocks: 8
Available Categories: 100
Allocated Categories: 72
Asterisk Categories: 6
Chapter Type: Body System Chapter

Introduction to the chapter

This chapter covers diseases of the skin and subcutaneous tissue. There are 8 blocks assigned to this chapter. Many of the blocks and categories in this chapter have inclusions and some have long lists of exclusions with cross-references in parentheses. Note that there are 10 exclusions listed at the beginning of the chapter. Study them well before continuing; otherwise you will make serious errors in coding from this chapter.

Some common examples from this chapter are: skin abscesses, carbuncles & furuncles, impetigo, cellulites, pilonidal cyst, lymphadenitis, eczema, dermatitis, pruritis, psoriasis, urticaria, sunburn, alopecia, acne, vitiligo, corns & callosities, lupus erythematosus, and nail disorders.

Chapter-specific notes

1. Be careful in coding from block 1 of this chapter (L00-L08, infections of the skin and subcutaneous tissue), as many diseases in this block are coded to the site of the infection (distributed throughout Volume 1) and some local infections of the skin are classified in Chapter I, hence the many exclusions—both at the block and category levels.

2. Note that in the block including "dermatitis and eczema" (categories L20-L30), the terms "dermatitis" and "eczema" are used synonymously and interchangeably.

3. An additional external cause code (Chapter XX) may be used (if desired) with categories L23.3, L25.1, L27.0, and L27.1 (contact dermatitis due to drugs in contact with skin) to identify drug. The same applies for the category L93 (lupus erythematosus) if the condition is drug-induced.

Exercise 6.12

Circle either T (True) or F (False) for the following statements:

1. There are no exclusions listed at the beginning of this chapter.   T   F

2. Chapter I must be carefully considered while coding skin infections from block 1 of this chapter.   T   F

3. Nail disorders are not to be coded from this chapter.   T   F

4. There are 6 asterisk categories in this chapter.   T   F

5. This is not a body system chapter.   T   F

CODING EXERCISE – CHAPTER XII

I. Using Volume 3 (Index) of the ICD-10, provide appropriate codes for the following diagnostic statement:

No.	Diagnostic statements	ICD-10 code
1	Vitiligo	
2	Decubitus ulcer	
3	Acne tropica	
4	Mucinosis of skin	
5	Xerosis cutis	
6	Localized hypertrichosis	
7	Alopecia universalis	
8	Solar urticaria	
9	Lichen planus	
10	Psoriasis vulgaris	
11	Pruritis vulvae	
12	Seborrhea capitis	
13	Bullous pemphigoid	
14	Cellulitis of finger	
15	Onychogryphosis	
16	Acute radiodermatitis	
17	Linear scleroderma	
18	Keloid scar	
19	Bockhart's impetigo	
20	Pemphigus vegetans	

II. Using Volume 1 (Four-Character Categories, Tabular List),
provide *complete* diagnostic statements for the following codes:

No.	ICD-10 code	Diagnostic statement
1	L70.0	
2	L60.0	
3	L50.6	
4	L40.1	
5	L03.2	

CHAPTER XIII

Title: Diseases of the Musculoskeletal System and Connective Tissue

> Range of Codes: M00-M99
> Number of Blocks: 6
> Available Categories: 100
> Allocated Categories: 79
> Asterisk Categories: 12
> Chapter Type: Body System Chapter

Introduction to the chapter

This chapter covers diseases and conditions relating to the spine, joints, muscles and connective tissue of the body. It also covers deformities acquired after birth. There are nine exclusions to be taken note of at the beginning of this chapter as well as those at the block and category levels. The chapter is made up of six major blocks, four of which are broken down into smaller sub-blocks. Before studying the blocks of this chapter, look at the section entitled "Site of musculoskeletal involvement" which you will find on the second page of this chapter. This is an additional, optional sub classification provided to indicate the site of involvement where appropriate. Further supplementary classifications for optional use are given at a) M23 (internal derangement of knee), M25 (other joint disorders), b) M40-M54 (Dorsopathies, except M50, M51), c) M60-M66 (disorders of muscles), and d) M99 (Biomechanical lesions).

Some common examples from this chapter are: arthritis, gout, spondylitis, disc problems, sciatica, lumbago, backache, myositis, sprains & strains, osteomyelitis, bursitis, synovitis, tendonitis, etc.

Chapter-specific notes

1. Apply caution while coding from the block entitled "Disorders of muscles" (M60-M63) which includes inflammation, wasting and calcification of the muscle: keep in mind that if the muscle disorder is caused by an injury, it is classified within chapter XIX—Injury & poisoning & consequences of external causes:

2. Category M99 (Biomechanical lesions) should not be used if the condition can be classified elsewhere.

3. In categories M15-M19 the term "osteoarthritis" is used as a synonym for "arthrosis" or "osteoarthritis".

Exercise 6.13

Circle either T (True) or F (False) where appropriate.

1. This is a special chapter.		T	F
2. "Low back pain" can be coded from this chapter.		T	F
3. Dorsopathies are provided with an additional, optional sub classification of site.		T	F
4. If a muscle disorder is caused by an injury it should be classified within chapter XIX.		T	F
5. This chapter has 65 allocated categories.		T	F

I. Using Volume 3 (Index) of the ICD-10, provide appropriate codes for the following diagnostic statement:

No.	Diagnostic statements	ICD-10 code
1	Juvenile rheumatoid arthritis	
2	Flat foot, acquired	
3	Postural kyphosis	
4	Infantile idiopathic scoliosis	
5	Adult osteochondrosis of spine	
6	Spinal stenosis	
7	Pott's curvature	
8	Infective myositis	
9	Low back pain	
10	Calcific tendonitis	
11	Contracture of muscle	
12	Muscle strain	
13	Prepatellar bursitis	
14	Rupture of synovium	
15	Achilles tendonitis	
16	Osteoporosis of disuse	
17	Senile osteomalacia	
18	Acquired deformity of nose	
19	Reiter's disease	
20	Gout due to renal impairment	

II. Using Volume 1 (Four-Character Categories, Tabular List), provide *complete* diagnostic statements for the following codes:

No.	ICD-10 code	Diagnostic statement
1	M45	
2	M70.1	
3	M81.0	
4	M06.9	
5	M86.2	

CHAPTER XIV

Title: **Diseases of the Genitourinary System**

Range of Codes: N00-N99
Number of Blocks: 11
Available Categories: 100
Allocated Categories: 82
Asterisk Categories: 9
Chapter Type: Body System Chapter

Introduction to the chapter

This chapter covers the urinary system and the male and female reproductive organs. In total there are 11 blocks, the first six of them devoted to the urinary system, the next block covering the diseases of the male genital organs, the following block dealing with the disorders of breast, the next two blocks dealing with the diseases of the female genital organs and the last block (N99) covering other disorders of the genito-urinary system. At the beginning of the first block (N00-N08, Glomerular diseases) there is a list of standardized fourth-character subdivisions (.0 to .9), for use with N00-N07, to indicate morphological changes when identified by renal biopsy or autopsy. Use these with the 3-digit categories relating to the clinical syndromes.

Important examples from this chapter are: nephritis, renal failure, renal calculi, prostate disorders, male & female infertility, menstrual disorders, uterine disorders, cystitis, etc.

Chapter-specific notes

1. Disorders of the breast usually occur in the female, however, these conditions *can* occur in the male as well, so don't be misled when you come across this block (Disorders of breast, N60-N64) while coding.

2. Categories N00-N07 relate to glomerular dysfunctions as well defined clinical syndromes. There is provision for a fourth-character subdivision (ranging from .0 to .9) for classifying morphological changes. However, these should not normally be used unless specifically identified by renal biopsy or autopsy.

3. For categories N17-N19 (Renal failure) an external cause code (Chapter XX) may be used, if desired, to identify the external agent.

Exercise 6.14

Fill in the blank spaces in the following statement:

Chapter XIV has .... blocks, the first .... of them are concerned with the urinary system; the next block covers the diseases of the .... genital organs, the next one deals with the disorders of ...., the following .... blocks covering disorders of the female .... system; and the last block (N ....) covering other disorders of the genitourinary system.

I. Using Volume 3 (Index) of the ICD-10, provide appropriate codes
for the following diagnostic statement:

No.	Diagnostic statements	ICD-10 code
1	Inversion of uterus	
2	Chronic obstructive pyelonephritis	
3	Acute renal failure with medullary necrosis	
4	Primary amenorrhea	
5	Female sterility associated with anovulation	
6	Post procedural renal failure	
7	Endometriosis of uterus	
8	Acute vaginitis	
9	Cyst of Bartholin's gland	
10	Atrophy of prostate	
11	Impotence of organic origin	
12	Infected hydrocele	
13	Atrophy of breast	
14	Chronic salpingitis	
15	Male sterility	
16	Polyp of vulva	
17	Primary oligomenorrhea	
18	Premenstrual tension syndrome	
19	Nonspecific urethritis	
20	Stress incontinence	

II. Using Volume 1 (Four-Character Categories, Tabular List), provide *complete* diagnostic statements for the following codes:

No.	ICD-10 code	Diagnostic statement
1	N71.0	
2	N80.1	
3	N97.1	
4	N17.0	
5	N40	

CHAPTER XV

Title: Pregnancy Childbirth & the Puerperium

Range of Codes: O00-O99
Number of Blocks: 8
Available Categories: 100
Allocated Categories: 75
Asterisk Categories: None
Chapter Type: Special Chapter

Introduction to the chapter

This chapter covers disorders and complications that arise during pregnancy, childbirth and the puerperium (the period following delivery). For statistical purposes, events within 42 days of delivery are considered to be within the puerperal period. There are 8 blocks in total, which follow the progress of pregnancy through to the end of the puerperium period. The first three blocks are mostly concerned with pregnancy, the next three blocks cover delivery and complications of delivery, the following block covers the puerperium (including lactation problems), and the last block covers other conditions which complicate pregnancy & childbirth that have not been classified elsewhere (including maternal death).

Common disorders of this chapter include ectopic pregnancy, abortion, placenta praevia, antepartum haemorrhage, long labour, delivery, malposition & malpresentation of fetus, puerperal sepsis, breast disorders, and maternal death.

Chapter-specific notes

1. Coders will frequently encounter such diagnoses (especially at the primary healthcare level) as antenatal care or supervision of normal (or high risk) pregnancy. At such times they should consult Chapter XXI ("Factors influencing health status") instead of this chapter and find the relevant code (Z34 or Z35).

2. Categories O03-O06 are three-digit categories that deal with spontaneous, medical, or other types of abortions. Coders are expected to add the fourth digits for these categories from a list of subdivisions ranging (from .0 to .9) provided at the beginning of the chapter.

3. Categories O20-O29 deal with maternal disorders predominantly related to pregnancy. However, two categories (i.e. O24.- Diabetes mellitus in pregnancy, and O25, Malnutrition in pregnancy) can be used even if they occur during childbirth or the puerperium.

4. Codes O80-O84 (Delivery) are provided for morbidity purposes. Codes from these categories should be used for primary morbidity coding only if no other condition classifiable to this chapter (i.e. Chapter XV) is recorded.

5. Categories O88.- (Obstetric embolism), O91.- (Infections of breast associated with childbirth), and 092.- (Other disorders of breast and lactation associated with childbirth) indicate complications predominantly related to the puerperium. However, these codes may be used even if the conditions listed there occur during pregnancy and childbirth.

6. Categories O95-O97 list obstetric conditions, not elsewhere classified, but before using these categories the coder should refer to the mortality coding rules and guidelines in Volume 2.

Exercise 6.15

Fill in the blank spaces in the following statements:

> Chapter XV has .... Blocks. The first .... blocks are concerned with pregnancy, the next three blocks cover .... and its complications; the following block covers the .... (including .... problems), and the .... block covers other conditions, which complicate .... & childbirth.

CODING EXERCISE – CHAPTER XV

I. Using Volume 3 (Index) of the ICD-10, provide appropriate codes
for the following diagnostic statement:

No.	Diagnostic statements	ICD-10 code
1	Spontaneous breech delivery	
2	Missed abortion	
3	Multiple pregnancy	
4	Malformation of placenta	
5	Pre-term delivery	
6	Obstructed labor due to locked twins	
7	Postpartum coagulation defects	
8	Infection of obstetric surgical wound	
9	Maternal care for cervical incompetence	
10	Delivery by emergency cesarean section	
11	Antepartum hemorrhage with coagulation defect	
12	Placenta previa without hemorrhage	
13	Threatened abortion	
14	Hemorrhoids in pregnancy	
15	Infections of bladder in pregnancy	
16	Low forceps delivery	
17	Pyrexia during labor	
18	Galactorrhea	
19	Anemia complicating pregnancy	
20	Abdominal pregnancy	

II. Using Volume 1 (Four-Character Categories, Tabular List), provide *complete* diagnostic statements for the following codes:

No.	ICD-10 code	Diagnostic statement
1	O69.0	
2	O91.1	
3	O15.1	
4	O04.2	
5	O03.9	

CHAPTER XVI

Title: Certain Conditions Originating in the Perinatal Period

Range of Codes: P00-P96
Number of Blocks: 10
Available Categories: 97
Allocated Categories: 59
Asterisk Categories: 1
Chapter Type: Special Chapter

Introduction to the chapter

Chapter XVI is concerned with conditions affecting the fetus and the newborn baby originating in the perinatal period. The perinatal period begins at 22 completed weeks (154 days) of gestation (the time when birth weight is normally 500g), and ends seven completed days after birth. As with other chapters in ICD-10, exclusions are frequently listed throughout the chapter, however, the relevant category is always given. Disorders related to length of gestation and fetal growth (P05-P08) cover situations where the relationship between weight and gestation length is not as normally expected. Glossary type definitions are provided for disorders relating to the length of gestation and fetal growth.

Common examples of this chapter are: birth trauma, gestational disorders, intrauterine anoxia & hypoxia, birth asphyxia, respiratory distress syndrome of newborn, and perinatal infections.

Chapter-specific notes

1. Be careful in coding from this and the previous chapter (Chapter XV). Often coders select a code for maternal care related to the fetus (O30-O48) from this chapter. This chapter covers *only those conditions that*

originate in the perinatal period and cause fetal death or morbidity, either during the perinatal period or later.

2. Categories P35-P39 provide codes for infections acquired in utero or during birth and they are specific only to the perinatal period. For any other infections the coder must look to other chapters, as guided.

Exercise 6.16

Fill in the blank spaces in the following statement:

The perinatal period begins at .... completed weeks

(...............days) of gestation (the time when birth weight is normally

.......................g), and ends .... completed days

after ....

CODING EXERCISE – CHAPTER XVI

I. Using Volume 3 (Index) of the ICD-10, provide appropriate codes for the following diagnostic statement:

No.	Diagnostic statements	ICD-10 code
1	Fetal death	
2	Meconium plug syndrome	
3	Noninfective neonatal diarrhea	
4	Coma of the newborn	
5	Umbilical polyp of newborn	
6	Dehydration of newborn	
7	Urinary tract infection of the newborn	
8	Respiratory failure of newborn	
9	Cold injury syndrome	
10	Aspiration of blood from newborn	
11	Congenital pneumonia due to pseudomonas	
12	Intrauterine hypoxia	
13	Birth injury to spleen	
14	Sepsis of newborn due to streptococcus, group B	
15	Fetal blood loss from placenta	
16	Neonatal hematemesis	
17	ABO isoimmunization of fetus and newborn	
18	Hydrops fetalis due to isoimmunization	
19	Neonatal jaundice due to polycythemia	
20	Kernicterus due to isoimmunization	

II. Using Volume 1 (Four-Character Categories, Tabular List), provide *complete* diagnostic statements for the following codes:

No.	ICD-10 code	Diagnostic statement
1	P07.2	
2	P37.5	
3	P00.5	
4	P22.0	
5	P90	

CHAPTER XVII

Title: Congenital Malformations, Deformations and Chromosomal Abnormalities

> Range of Codes: Q00-Q99
> Number of Blocks: 11
> Available Categories: 100
> Allocated Categories: 87
> Asterisk Categories: None
> Chapter Type: Special Chapter

Introduction to the chapter

This chapter covers all types of congenital malformations, deformations and chromosomal anomalies. It has 11 blocks, each covering a different body system. Included in these chapters are those anomalies resulting in visible structural malformations. Anomalies, which can be identified only by laboratory or chemical analysis, are assigned to other chapters. For example, inborn errors of metabolism are classified in Chapter IV (Endrocrine, nutritional, and metabolic diseases).

Some commonly occurring disorders from this chapter are: anencephaly, microcephaly, spina bifida, cleft palate & lip, undescended testicle, hypospadias, polydactyly & syndactyly; Down's, Turner's & Klinefelter's syndromes; hermaphroditism, etc.

Chapter specific notes

1. Certain metabolic disorders are decidedly congenital in nature (e.g. phenylketonuria, albinism, alkaptonuria, lactose intolerance, cystic fibrosis, etc.) and you might be tempted to classify these from this chapter. If you did this you would be committing an error. The codes for these conditions would be found in chapter IV (Endocrine,

nutritional and metabolic diseases). There are many such instances, so be careful in reading the *exclusion notes* well.

2. While coding "cleft lip and cleft palate" (categories Q35-Q37) from this chapter an additional code, Q30.2 ("Fissured, notched and cleft nose) may also be used, if desired, to identify associated malformations of the nose.

Exercise 6.17

Circle either T (True) or F (False) in the following statements:

1. This chapter has no asterisk categories.	T	F
2. Inborn errors of metabolism are classified in chapter IV.	T	F
3. You can code cystic fibrosis from this chapter.	T	F
4. The code for Down's syndrome exists in this chapter.	T	F
5. This chapter has 87 available categories.	T	F

CODING EXERCISE – CHAPTER XVII

I. Using Volume 3 (Index) of the ICD-10, provide appropriate codes
for the following diagnostic statements:

No.	Diagnostic statements	ICD-10 code
1	Down's syndrome	
2	Fragile X chromosome	
3	Spina bifida occulta	
4	Osteogenesis imperfecta	
5	Xeroderma pigmentosum	
6	Conjoined twins	
7	Klinefelter's syndrome	
8	Congenital deformity of knee	
9	Renal dysplasia	
10	Displacement of ureter	
11	Marfan's syndrome	
12	Undescended testicle, unilateral	
13	Perineal hypospadias	
14	Atresia of bile ducts	
15	Cleft lip, unilateral	
16	Web of larynx	
17	Ventricular septal defect	
18	Tetralogy of Fallot	
19	Arnold-Chiari syndrome	
20	Patent ductus arteriosus	

II. Using Volume 1 (Four-Character Categories, Tabular List), provide
complete diagnostic statements for the following codes:

No.	ICD-10 code	Diagnostic statement
1	Q35.1	
2	Q03.8	
3	Q98.0	
4	Q13.3	
5	Q65.1	

CHAPTER XVIII

Title: Symptoms, Signs and Abnormal Clinical and Laboratory Findings, Not Elsewhere Classified.

Range of Codes: R00-R99
Number of Blocks: 13
Available Categories: 100
Allocated Categories: 90
Asterisk Categories: None
Chapter Type: General Chapter

Introduction to the chapter

This chapter covers symptoms, signs and abnormal results of clinical or other investigative procedures. It also includes ill-defined conditions regarding which no diagnosis classifiable elsewhere is recorded. In general, categories in this chapter cover the less well-defined conditions and symptoms that, without the necessary study of the case, could point equally to more than one disease, or more than one body system. The chapter is divided into 13 blocks, eight of which refer to symptoms and signs involving various systems. The next four blocks relate to abnormal findings and the last block refers to ill defined and unknown causes of mortality (e.g. sudden infant death syndrome, unknown cause of mortality).

Some common examples from this chapter are: nosebleed, heartburn, cramps, painful urination, drowsiness, headache, fever of unknown origin, cough, nausea and vomiting, malaise & fatigue, dizziness, etc.

Chapter-specific notes

1. Categories from this chapter should *NOT* be used as main conditions unless the symptom, sign or abnormal finding is the *only* diagnosis recorded by the doctor. If a more precise or definite diagnosis is

recorded, make attempts to find the suitable code from another, appropriate chapter.

2. Categories R83-R89 are made up of three-character codes for abnormal findings on examination of other body fluids, substances and tissues, without diagnosis. Four-character subdivisions (ranging from .0 to .9) are provided at the beginning of this block of categories for use to identify the precise abnormality (e.g. .0 "Abnormal level of enzymes"; .1 "Abnormal level of hormones", etc.).

Exercise 6.18

Use the words given on the left to complete the statement on the right.

appropriate ⎫	Signs and .... pointing to a ....
symptoms ⎪	
definite ⎬	diagnosis will have been .... to a
assigned ⎭	
	category in the .... chapter.

CODING EXERCISE – CHAPTER XVIII

I. Using Volume 3 (Index) of the ICD-10, provide appropriate codes for the following diagnostic statement:

No.	Diagnostic statements	ICD-10 code
1	Restlessness	
2	Persistent fever	
3	Headache	
4	Chronic intractable pain	
5	Febrile convulsions	
6	Lymphadenopathy	
7	Abnormal weight loss	
8	Ataxic gait	
9	Meningismus	
10	Painful urination	
11	Finding of cocaine in blood	
12	Abnormality of red blood cells	
13	Isolated proteinuria	
14	Abnormal glucose tolerance test	
15	Unattended death	
16	Glycosuria	
17	Generalized edema	
18	Hypovolemic shock	
19	Auditory hallucination	
20	Extrarenal uremia	

II. Using Volume 1 (Four-Character Categories, Tabular List), provide *complete* diagnostic statements for the following codes:

No.	ICD-10 code	Diagnostic statement
1	R95	
2	R59.0	
3	R46.0	
4	R94.4	
5	R04.1	

CHAPTER XIX

**Title: Injury, Poisoning and Certain other Consequences of
External Causes**

Range of Codes: S00-T98
Number of Blocks: 21
Available Categories: 199
Allocated Categories: 195
Asterisk Categories: None
Chapter Type: Special Chapter

Introduction to the chapter

This chapter classifies the *nature* of the injury or other effects of external causes. It may conveniently be divided into four major groups. The first and second groups deal with injuries and poisonings, respectively. The third group lists complications of surgical and medical care, and the last group is concerned with sequelae of injuries and poisoning. The "sequelae" include those specified as such, as late effects, and those, which are present one year or more after the acute injury. For coding different types of injuries, this chapter lists ten "body regions" (head, neck, thorax, etc.), each being allocated ten three-character categories, which follow a similar pattern (i.e. superficial injury, open wound, fracture, dislocation, etc.)

Chapter-specific notes

1. Be guided by the fact that this chapter uses the "S" section for coding different types of injuries related to *single* body regions and the "T" section to cover injuries to *multiple* or unspecified body regions as well as poisoning. Also, make sure that you do not use codes T90-T98 (sequelae of injuries & poisoning) as main conditions if the nature of the residual conditions is recorded.

2. Where multiple sites of injury are specified in the titles, the word "with" indicates involvement of both sites, and the word "and" indicates involvement of either or both sides.

3. Use additional external cause code (Chapter XX) to identify the corresponding cause or devices involved and details of circumstances.

4. There is provision in this chapter for a fifth-character sub division (represented by 0 and 1) to indicate open and closed fractures as well as intracranial, intrathoracic and intra-abdominal injuries with and without open wound. Thus "open" and "closed" fracture of hip (S72.0) could be coded as S72.01 and S72.00, respectively. Note that a fracture not indicated as open or closed should be classified as closed, (i. e. 0).

5. Category T31 ("Burns classified according to extent of body surface involved") is to be used as the primary code only when the site of the burn is unspecified. It may be used as a supplementary code, if desired, with categories T20-T29 when the site is specified.

Exercise 6.19

Circle either T (True) or F (False) against the following statements:

1. This chapter is a body system chapter.		T	F
2. The "T" section of this chapter covers injuries to multiple or unspecified body regions as well as to poisoning.		T	F
3. The sequelae of injuries include injuries that are present one year or more after the acute injury.		T	F
4. This chapter deals with the nature of the injury.		T	F
5. This chapter includes 195 asterisk categories.		T	F

CODING EXERCISE – CHAPTER XIX

I. Using Volume 3 (Index) of the ICD-10, provide appropriate codes for the following diagnostic statements:

No.	Diagnostic statement	ICD-10 code
1	Open wound of knee	
2	Dislocation of hip	
3	Crushing injury of hip with thigh	
4	Heat exhaustion	
5	Psychological abuse	
6	Traumatic shock	
7	Rh incompatibility reaction	
8	Injury of popliteal vein	
9	Contusion of knee	
10	Open wound of abdominal wall	
11	Burn of third degree of wrist and hand	
12	Frostbite with tissue necrosis of neck	
13	Poisoning by sulfonamides	
14	Epidural hemorrhage	
15	Concussion	
16	Burns involving 50-59% of unspecified site of body surface	
17	Superficial frostbite of arm	
18	Poisoning by local anesthetics	
19	Toxic effect of hydrogen sulfide	
20	Motion sickness	

II. Using Volume 1 (Four-Character Categories, Tabular List), provide *complete* diagnostic statements for the following codes:

No.	ICD-10 code	Diagnostic statement
1	S22.3	
2	T53.1	
3	T17.4	
4	T01.0	
5	T65.2	

CHAPTER XX

Title: External Causes of Morbidity and Mortality

Range of Codes: V01-Y98
Number of Blocks: 8
Available Categories: 399
Allocated Categories: 372
Asterisk Categories: None
Chapter Type: External Chapter

Introduction to the chapter

This chapter permits the classification of external events and circumstances as the cause of injury, poisoning and other adverse effects. It is intended that, where a code from this chapter is applicable, it should normally be used together with a code from another chapter giving the *nature* of the injury or condition (Chapter XIX)

This chapter is the largest in ICD-10 using four letters V, W, X, and Y. *Accidents* (V01-X59) constitute a major portion of this chapter followed by suicide attempts, assault, and others. There is a "place of occurrence" code to be used as a fourth character subdivision with categories W00-Y34 (except Y06.- and Y07.-) to identify the place of occurrence of the accident where relevant. There is also a provision for "activity codes" for optional use in a supplementary character position, with categories V01-Y34. They are used to indicate the activity of the injured person at the time the event occurred.

Chapter-specific notes

1. The codes for external causes (V01-Y89) should be used in addition to a code from Chapter XIX (injury & poisoning). Causes of death should preferably be tabulated according to both Chapters XIX and Chapter XX, but if only one code is tabulated then the code from Chapter XX should be used in preference.

2. Don't forget to use Section II ("External causes of injury") and Section III ("Table of drugs and chemicals") of the Index in coding the external causes of injuries and poisonings.

3. Most codes from this chapter are three-character codes followed by point and dash (.-) and hence incomplete. You must provide the fourth character by using the "place of occurrence" list at the beginning of the chapter. It ranges from .0 ("home") to .9 ("unspecified place").

Exercise 6.20

Fill in the blank spaces to make the following statements complete.

The codes for external causes (...... .-Y89) should be used together with a code from chapter .... Causes of death should preferably be coded from both chapters: Chapter .... and Chapter .... , but if only .... code is to be tabulated then the code from Chapter .... should be used in preference.

CODING EXERCISE – CHAPTER XX

I. Using Volume 1 and Volume 3 of the ICD-10, provide appropriate codes for the following diagnostic statements:

NOTE: Use "Place of Occurrence" code at the fourth-character level for these accidents.

No.	Diagnostic statement	ICD-10 code
1	Exposure to X-ray radiation, in hospital	
2	Strangulation by pillow, in hotel	
3	Victim of volcanic eruption, at mountain	
4	Bitten by dog, on road	
5	War operations involving land mine explosion	
6	Car accident	
7	Burn by hotplate, at home	
8	Legal intervention involving gas	
9	Run over by machinery, at farm	
10	Choked on bone, at restaurant	
11	Cutting misadventure during heart catheterization	
12	Asphyxia from forest fire	
13	Obstruction of esophagus by vomitus, at home	
14	Collapse of burning building, at factory	
15	Drowning in bathtub, at home	
16	Motion sickness, at motorway	
17	Intentional self-harm by sleeping pills	
18	Mismatched blood in transfusion	
19	Accidental poisoning by lead acetate	
20	Adverse effect of penicillin in therapeutic use	

II. Using Volume 1 (Four-Character Categories, Tabular List), provide *complete* diagnostic statements for the following codes:

No.	ICD-10 code	Diagnostic statement
1	V87.3	
2	W05.2	
3	W53.0	
4	X72.9	
5	X45.9	

CHAPTER XXI

Title: Factors Influencing Health Status and Contact with Health Services

Range of Codes: Z00-Z99
Number of Blocks: 7
Available Categories: 100
Allocated Categories: 84
Asterisk Categories: None
Chapter Type: External Chapter

Introduction to the chapter

This chapter is provided for occasions when circumstances other than a disease, injury or external cause classifiable to chapters I-XX are recorded as "diagnoses" or "problems". This applies when one of the following occurs:

1. A person who may or may not be sick encounters the health services for some specific service which is not related to a disease or injury, for example, bringing a child for vaccination, discussion of a problem, etc.

2. Some circumstance or problem is present which influences the person's health status but is not in itself a current illness or injury: for example, artificial limb, dependent on wheel chair, presence of artificial eye, etc.

3. The chapter is divided into seven blocks. There are important notes at the beginning of most blocks, which should be carefully read.

Chapter-specific notes

This chapter is for use in *morbidity coding only* and must not be used for international comparison or for primary mortality coding.

Exercise 6.21

Put ✓ against those conditions that can be coded from this chapter and ✗ against those whose code must be found elsewhere.

1. Malnutrition ....
2. Lack of adequate food ....
3. Emotional neglect of child ....
4. Antenatal screening ....
5. Personal history of leukaemia ....
6. Leukaemia ....
7. Diabetes mellitus ....
8. Family history of diabetes mellitus ....
9. Tobacco use ....
10. Drug dependence ....

CODING EXERCISE – CHAPTER XXI

I. Using Volume 3 (Index) of the ICD-10, provide appropriate codes for the following diagnostic statements:

No.	Diagnostic statement	ICD-10 code
1	Supervision of normal first pregnancy	
2	Prophylactic vaccination against smallpox	
3	Carrier of viral hepatitis	
4	Screening for neoplasm of breast	
5	Laboratory examination	
6	Observation for suspected tuberculosis	
7	Contraceptive management	
8	Genetic counseling	
9	Personal history of allergy to penicillin	
10	Family history of diabetes mellitus	
11	Acquired absence of foot and ankle	
12	Occupational health examination	
13	Issue of medical certificate	
14	Confirmed pregnancy	
15	Follow-up examination following psychotherapy	
16	Medical examination for driving license	
17	Fertility test	
18	Fitting of external breast prosthesis	
19	Insertion of intrauterine contraceptive device	
20	Medical examination for insurance purposes	

II. Using Volume 1 (Four-Character Categories, Tabular List), provide *complete* diagnostic statements for the following codes:

No.	ICD-10 code	Diagnostic statement
1	Z94.5	
2	Z01.2	
3	Z99.3	
4	Z00.1	
5	Z35.9	

CHAPTER XXII

Title: Codes for Special Purposes

Range of Codes: U00-U99
Number of Blocks: 2 (only 1 specified so far)
Available Categories: 100
Allocated Categories: 1
Asterisk Categories: None
Chapter Type: Special Chapter

Introduction to the chapter

The unused "U" codes of the First Edition of ICD-10 have been incorporated in a new Chapter (Chapter XXII) in the Second Edition of ICD-10. There are two major blocks into which the new codes are to be accommodated. Codes within the first block (U00-U49) are to be used for the provisional assignment of new diseases of uncertain etiology. Codes belonging to the second block (U50-U99) may be used in research, e.g. when testing an alternative sub classification for a specific project. The Second Edition of ICD-10 shows one three-character category (U04, severe acute respiratory syndrome, SARS), and its four-character subdivision (U04.9, severe acute respiratory syndrome, unspecified) within the first block. The second block is still unused. It is anticipated that future editions of ICD-10 shall have more codes assigned to this chapter.

Exercise 6.22

Fill in the blanks spaces:

The title of Chapter XXII is "Codes for ....

It has been assigned a total of 100 codes (U00-U99). Codes U00-U49 are to be

used for the .... assignment of new diseases of uncertain

.... Codes U50-U.... may be used in ....

UNIT 7
MORBIDITY CODING

UNIT 7
MORBIDITY CODING

Overview of morbidity coding

For the purpose of ICD, the term morbidity covers illnesses, injuries, and reasons for contact with health services including screening and preventive care. Coding usually relates to an episode of health care but may also apply to health surveys. An episode of health care is either:

    a) a period of inpatient care, or

    b) a contact with a health care practitioner in relation to the same condition or its immediate consequences.

There are many sources for morbidity data, such as hospital records, primary care records, school health records, armed services records, and health surveys. Some other sources are outpatient records, records of maternal & child health services, cancer and chronic disease registry records, etc.

There are many uses for morbidity data. Such data may provide clues to the causes of disease. It may also form the basis on which decisions are made about preventive measures or the allocation of resources.

Central concepts of morbidity coding

At the end of an episode of health care the attending health care practitioner ideally records *all* the conditions, which affected the patient. This does not mean that the coder should codify all the conditions so listed. Coding one condition from the case notes is called "single-condition coding" and coding all conditions is called "multiple condition coding". Most establishment use *single-condition coding* either because the lack of resources restricts coders to one condition only, or the simpler data provided by *single condition coding* may be more appropriate for the establishment's needs.

Whatever the reasons for using single-condition coding, the rules are the same. One of the conditions recorded on the case notes must be selected as the "main condition". The **main condition** *is the condition diagnosed, at the end of the episode of health care, primarily responsible for the patient receiving treatment or being investigated.* In other words, the main condition is the condition diagnosed as being primarily responsible for the episode of health care.

Normally, accompanying conditions should also be coded. They are known as other conditions. **Other conditions** are *those conditions that co-exist or develop during the episode of health care and affect the management of the patient.*

Often the physicians put down one of the *other* conditions as the *main* condition. If that happens, your first course of action as a coder must be to refer the case record back to the physician. Usually it would be returned with the main condition reselected or some clarification will be given (See Figure 1).

Failing this, and only as a last resort, you should apply the *reselection rules* MB1 to MB5. These are explained as follows:

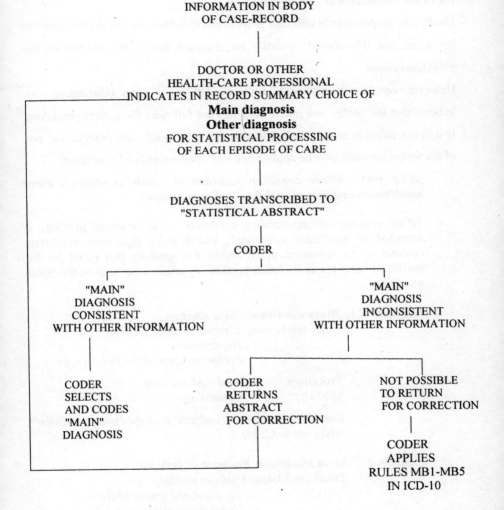

INFORMATION IN BODY
OF CASE-RECORD

DOCTOR OR OTHER
HEALTH-CARE PROFESSIONAL
INDICATES IN RECORD SUMMARY CHOICE OF
Main diagnosis
Other diagnosis
FOR STATISTICAL PROCESSING
OF EACH EPISODE OF CARE

DIAGNOSES TRANSCRIBED TO
"STATISTICAL ABSTRACT"

CODER

"MAIN"
DIAGNOSIS
CONSISTENT
WITH OTHER INFORMATION

"MAIN"
DIAGNOSIS
INCONSISTENT
WITH OTHER INFORMATION

CODER
SELECTS
AND CODES
"MAIN"
DIAGNOSIS

CODER
RETURNS
ABSTRACT
FOR CORRECTION

NOT POSSIBLE
TO RETURN
FOR CORRECTION

CODER
APPLIES
RULES MB1-MB5
IN ICD-10

Figure 1

Rules for reselection of "main condition"

Ideally, the responsible health care practitioner indicates the "main condition" to be coded and this should normally be accepted for coding, subject to the guidelines above.

However, certain circumstances or the availability of other information may indicate that the health care practitioner has not followed the correct procedure. If it is not possible to obtain clarification from the health care practitioner, one of the following rules may be applied and the "main condition" reselected.

RULE MB1. Minor condition recorded as "main condition", more significant condition recorded as "other condition".

Where a minor or long-standing condition, or an incidental problem, is recorded as the "main condition", and a more significant condition, relevant to the treatment given and/or the specialty that cared for the patient, is recorded as an "other condition", reselect the latter as the "main condition".

Example 1: **Main condition**: *Acute sinusitis*
Other conditions: *Carcinoma of endocervix*
Hypertension
Patient in hospital for three weeks

Procedure: *Total hysterectomy*
Specialty: *Gynecology*

Reselect *carcinoma of endocervix* as the "main condition"
And code to C53.0.

Example 2 **Main condition:** *Rheumatoid arthritis*
Other conditions: *Diabetes mellitus*
Strangulated femoral hernia
Generalized arteriosclerosis
Patient in hospital for two weeks

Procedure: *Herniorrhaphy*
Specialty: *Surgery*

Reselect *strangulated femoral hernia* as the "main condition" and code to K41.3.

RULE MB2. Several conditions recorded as "main condition"

If several conditions that cannot be coded together are recorded as the "main condition" and other details on the records point to one of them as being the "main condition", for which the patient received care, select that condition. Otherwise select the condition first mentioned.

Example 3: Main **condition**:   *Cataract*
                                  Staphylococcal meningitis
                                  Ischemic heart disease
              Other condition: -------
                                  Patient in hospital for five weeks
              Specialty: *Neurology*

Select *staphylococcal meningitis* as the "main condition" and code to G00.3.

Example 4: **Main condition:**   *Mitral stenosis*
                                  Acute bronchitis
                                  Rheumatoid arthritis

              Other condition: --------
              Specialty: *General medicine*

              No information about therapy.

              Select *mitral stenosis*, the first-mentioned condition, as the "main condition" and code to I05.0.

RULE MB3. Condition recorded as "main condition" is presenting symptom of diagnosed, treated condition.

If a symptom or sign (usually classifiable to Chapter XVIII), or a problem classifiable to Chapter XXI, is recorded as the "main condition" and this is obviously the presenting sign, symptom or problem of a diagnosed condition recorded elsewhere and care was given for the latter, reselect the diagnosed condition as the "main condition".

Example 5.   **Main condition:**   *Abdominal pain*
                  Other condition: *Acute appendicitis*
                   Procedure: *Appendectomy*

              Reselect *acute appendicitis* as the "main condition" and Code to K35.9.

Example 6:   **Main condition**: *Coma*
              Other conditions: *Ischaemic heart disease*
                                 Diabetes mellitus, insulin-dependent

              Specialty: *Endocrinology*
              Care: *Establishment of correct dose of*
                                 Insulin

Reselect *diabetes mellitus, insulin-dependent* as the
"main condition" and code to E10.0. The information
provided indicates that the coma was due to diabetes
mellitus and coma is taken into account as it modifies
the coding.

RULE MB4. Specificity

Where the diagnosis recorded as the "main condition" describes a
condition in general terms, and a term that provides more precise
information about the site or nature of the condition is recorded
elsewhere, reselect the latter as the "main condition".

Example 7   Main condition :   Cerebrovascular accident
              Other conditions: *Diabetes mellitus*
                                 Hypertension
                                 Cerebral haemorrhage

Reselect *cerebral haemorrhage* as the "main condition"
and code to I61.9

Example 8.   Main condition: *Congenital heart disease*
              Other conditions: *Ventricular septal defect*
              Reselect *ventricular septal defect* as the "main condition"
               and code to Q21.0.

RULE MB5. Alternative main diagnoses

Where a symptom or sign is recorded as the "main condition" with an
indication that it may be due to either one condition or another, select
the symptom as the "main condition". Where two or more conditions
are recorded as diagnostic options for the "main condition", select the
first condition recorded.

Example 9.   **Main condition**:   *Headache due to either stress and tension or acute sinusitis*

Other conditions: --------

Select *headache* as the "main condition" and code to R51.

Example 10.   **Main condition**:   *Acute cholecystitis or acute Pancreatitis*

Other conditions: --------

Select *acute cholecystitis* as the "main condition" and code to K81.0.

Other guidelines for morbidity coding

1. Encountering the dagger & asterisk code

Often you will find these two codes listed against the condition you are looking for. If applicable, both codes should be used since they denote two different pathways for a single condition. But if you must select only *one* code, choose the dagger code. For example:

Main condition: *Tuberculous pericarditis*
Other conditions: -------

Code to "*tuberculosis of other specified organs*" (A18.8✝) because tuberculosis is the original cause of pericarditis from the etiological angle. The asterisk code for *pericarditis* (I32.0*) may be used *optionally*.

2. Coding of unspecified conditions, symptoms and non-illness situations

If after an episode of health care, the main condition is still recorded as "suspected", "questionable", "unknown", etc., and there is no further information or clarification, the suspected diagnosis must be coded as if established, for example:

Main condition: *Suspected gastric ulcer*
Other conditions: -------

Code to K25.9, *gastric ulcer* as main condition.

2. Coding of external causes of morbidity

For injuries and other conditions due to external causes, both the *nature* of the condition and the *circumstances* of the external cause should be coded. The preferred "main condition" code should be that describing the *nature* of the condition. This will usually be classifiable to chapter XIX. The code from Chapter XX, indicating the *external cause* would be used as an optional additional code. But you are well advised to record this as well on the coding sheet. For example, suppose the patient file contains a case of a young boy sustaining an open wound of finger and thumb because of an accident caused by knife, accompanied by syncope and collapse. Your job as a coder would be not only to code the nature of the injury ("open wound of finger and thumb": *S61.0*) but also the external cause of injury ("Accident caused by knife": *W26.9*).

Main condition: *Open wound of finger & thumb (S61.0)*
Other condition: *Syncope and collapse (R55)*

The *External cause* code for "accident caused by knife" (W26.9) should also be used as an additional code.

Likewise if a patient arrives with a skull fracture and some minor skin cuts sustained in a car accident, the coding could be as follows:

Main condition: *Skull fracture (S02.9)*
Other condition: *Minor skin cuts* (T14.1)

The external cause code for car accident (V49.9) should also be used as an additional code.

Exercise 7   Fill in the blank spaces to make the statements complete.

1. The **Main Condition** is the condition .... at the .... of the .... of health care, ... responsible for the patient receiving treatment or being investigated.

2. **Other Conditions** are those conditions which .... or .... during the episode of health care and affect the .... of the patient.

3. According to Rule MB4 (Specificity), if the diagnosis recorded as the "main condition" describes a condition in .... terms, and a term that provides more .... information, reselect the .... as the " ....
condition".

UNIT 8
MORTALITY CODING

UNIT 8

MORTALITY CODING

Overview of Mortality Coding

The ICD has its origins in the preparation of mortality statistics. The main sources of mortality data are death certificates. Information on the death certificate may be provided by either a health care practitioner or, in the case of accidents or violent deaths, a coroner or a nationally designated official of the Medico-legal Department.

The person certifying the cause of death will enter the sequence of events leading to death on the death certificate in international format that is featured below:

INTERNATIONAL FORM OF MEDICAL CERTIFICATE OF CAUSE OF DEATH

<u>Cause of death</u>		Approximate interval between onset and death
I Disease or condition directly leading to death*	(a) .... due to (or as a consequence of)	....
Antecedent causes morbid conditions, if any, giving rise to the above cause, stating the underlying condition last	(b) .... due to (or as a consequence of) (c) .... due to (or as a consequence of) (d)	....
II Other significant conditions contributing to the death, but not related to the disease or condition causing it	....	....
*This does not mean the mode of dying, e.g. heart failure, respiratory failure. It means the disease, injury, or complication that caused death.		

It is recommended that a separate certificate should be used to record perinatal death. An international format is also recommended for this certificate. This is shown as under:

CERTIFICATE OF CAUSE OF PERINATAL DEATH

To be completed for stillbirths and live born infants dying within 168 hours (1 week) from birth

Identifying particulars
☐ This child was born live on   at   hours
        and died on   at   hours
☐ This child was stillborn on   at   hours
        and died before labour ☐ during labour ☐ not known ☐

Mother	Child

Date of birth ⬚⬚⬚⬚⬚ 1ˢᵗ day of last
or, if unknown age (years) ⬚ menstrual period ⬚⬚⬚⬚
   or if unknown estimated duration
Number of previous   of pregnancy ⬚
pregnancies: (completed weeks)
Live births ⬚
Still births ⬚
Abortions ⬚   Antenatal care, two or more visits:
   ☐ Yes
   ☐ No
Outcome of last previous   ☐ Not known
pregnancy:
☐ Live birth   Delivery:
☐ Stillbirth   ☐ Normal spontaneous vertex
☐ Abortion   other (specify)
Date ⬚⬚⬚⬚   ....
	Birthweight: .... Grams
	
	Sex: ☐ Boy ☐ Girl ☐ Indeterminate
	
	☐Single birth ☐ First twin
	
	☐Second twin ☐ Other multiple
	
	Attendant at birth
	☐ Physician ☐ Trained midwife
	Other trained person (specify)
	....
	Other (specify)
	....

Causes of death

a. Main disease or condition in fetus or infant

b. Other diseases or conditions in fetus or infant

c. Main maternal disease or condition affecting fetus or infant

d. Other maternal diseases or conditions affecting fetus or infant

e. Other relevant circumstances

| ☐ The certified cause of death has been confirmed
   by autopsy
☐ Autopsy information may be available later
☐ Autopsy not being held | I certify...............................
....
....

Signature and qualification |

Mortality data, in the form of ICD codes, is mainly used for the prevention of diseases and major causes of death after proper analysis. In fact once the data is collected, it is used like this:

DATA ⟶ ANALYSIS ⟶ RESOURCE MANAGEMENT ⟶ PREVENTION

The Concept of Underlying Cause

Many death certificates give only a single cause of death. These are relatively simple to deal with and all you have to do is code the single cause. However, in many cases, two or more morbid conditions contribute to death. These must all be recorded on the certificate. In such cases it has been the practice in Vital Statistics to select one of the causes of death for coding purposes. This single cause is usually given a special name -- the *underlying cause of death*. So, if you are coding a mortality case where there are several causes of death recorded, you will select one to be the underlying cause of death. The concept of the underlying cause of death is central to mortality coding. The underlying cause of death is defined as "the disease or injury which initiated the train of morbid events leading directly to death", or "the circumstances of the accident or violence which produced the fatal injury". In other words, the *underlying cause of death* is the condition, event or circumstance without which the patient would not have died. For example, suppose you are coding a cause where a cancer patient dies, and the immediate cause of death was *heart failure* resulting from carcinomatosis (spread of cancer), you might be tempted to assign heart failure as the underlying cause of death. This would be wrong. You may well be advised to reconsider the entire sequence of the morbid process as shown below:

Malignant bone cancer ⟶ carcinomatosis ⟶ heart failure ⟶ death

In this case, heart failure was the final morbid event in a sequence starting with bone cancer and thus the "direct cause" of death. "Malignant bone cancer" is the condition coded as the "underlying cause" of death.

It should be emphasized at this point that the responsibility for deciding on the logical sequence of death lies with the certifying doctor.

It is important that all deaths should be certified in the international format recommended by the W.H.O. The standard or International form of medical certificate of cause of death has two parts:

Part I: This is the main part of the certificate which is used for diseases related to the sequence of events leading *directly* to death.

Part II: This part is used for *unrelated* conditions which have no *direct* connection with events leading to death; but by their nature, contributed to death: diabetes, chronic asthma, ischemic heart disease, etc.

The certifying physician must ensure that the underlying cause of death is entered on the lowest used line in Part I. Also the coder must select the lowest entered condition as the underlying cause. Two other points must also be considered:

1. If death has occurred because of *injury*, it is the *external cause code* (Chapter XX) that should be used for single cause coding and tabulating underlying cause.

2. The asterisk (*) codes should not be used for coding mortality, as they are optional, additional codes. The dagger code (✝) is the primary code for this purpose.

General Principle and Rules

When *only* one cause of death is reported, this cause is used as the underlying cause of death. When *more than one* cause of death is recorded, the first step in selecting the underlying cause is to determine the originating antecedent cause proper, to the lowest used line in Part I of the certificate by application of the *General Principle* or of selection rules 1, 2, and 3.

In a properly filled certificate the originating cause will have been entered alone on the lowest used line of Part I and the conditions, if any that arose as a consequence of this initial cause will have been entered above it, one condition to a line in ascending causal order.

The following death certificate illustrates this process clearly. Although the patient eventually died of *uraemia* (or uraemic poisoning), the chain of morbid events had started much earlier, i.e. the patient's underlying problem was *hypertrophy* of *prostate*, which led to *urine retention* and *hydronephrosis* later. Because of these conditions, the patient developed uraemia, of which he died in the hospital. His other, or coexisting problems were *chronic asthma* and *old pulmonary tuberculosis*, but these conditions did not relate directly to *uraemia* which caused his death. The underlying cause of death, therefore, is "hypertrophy of prostate", coded as *N40* (Chapter XIV).

I	Cause of death	Approximate interval between onset and death
Disease or condition directly leading to death*	(a) ...*Uraemia*............ due to (or as a consequence of)	....
Antecedent causes morbid conditions, if any, giving rise to the above cause, stating the underlying condition last	(b) ...*Hydronephrosis*...... due to (or as a consequence of)	....
	(c) ...*Retention of urine*... due to (or as a consequence of)	....
II	(d) ...*Hypertrophy of prostate*	....
Other significant conditions contributing to the death, but not related to the disease or condition causing it	...*Chronic asthma*............ ...*Old pulmonary T.B*...	....

This does not mean the mode of dying, e.g. *heart failure, respiratory failure. It means the disease, injury, or complication that caused death.*

This kind of sequencing is used to formulate the *General Principle* that states that:

"When more than one condition is entered on the certificate, the condition entered alone on the lowest used line of Part I should be selected *only if it could have given rise to all the conditions entered above it*".

In a properly filled certificate, therefore, the *General Principle* will apply. But if the *General Principle* cannot be applied, clarification of the certificate should be sought from the certifier. Where further clarification cannot be obtained, however, the *selection rules* must be applied as illustrated below:

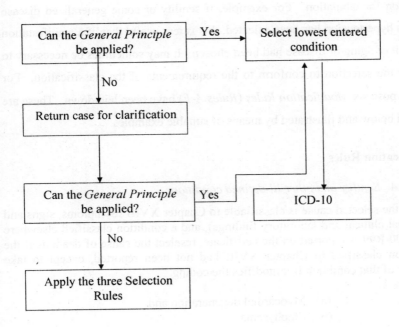

The three Selection Rules are stated as follows: -

Rule 1.   If the General Principle does not apply and there is a reported sequence terminating in the condition first entered on the certificate, select the originating cause of this sequence. *If there is more than one sequence terminating in the condition mentioned first, select the originating cause of the first-mentioned sequence.*

Rule 2.   If there is no reported sequence terminating in the condition first entered on the certificate, select this first-mentioned condition.

Rule 3.   If the condition selected by the General Principle, or by Rule 1 or Rule 2, is obviously a direct consequence of another reported condition, whether in Part I or Part II, select this primary condition.

Modification of the selected cause

The entered cause of death is not necessarily the most useful and informative condition for tabulation. For example, if senility or some generalized disease such as hypertension has been selected, this is less useful than if a manifestation or result of aging or disease had been chosen. It may sometimes be necessary to modify the selection to conform to the requirements of the classification. For this purpose six *Modification Rules* (*Rules A-F*) have been laid down. These are defined below and illustrated by means of suitable examples.

Modification Rules

RULE A. Senility and other ill-defined conditions

Where the selected cause is classifiable to Chapter XVIII (Symptoms, signs and abnormal clinical and laboratory findings), and a condition classified elsewhere than R00-R99 is reported on the certificate, reselect the cause of death as if the condition classified to Chapter XVIII had not been reported, except to take account of that condition if it modifies the coding.
Example 1:

  I   (a)   Myocardial degeneration and
         (b)   Emphysema
         (c)   Senility

Code to *myocardial degeneration* (I51.5). Senility, selected by the General Principle, is ignored and Rule 2 applied.

Example 2:

> I (a) Cough and haematemesis
>
> Code to *haematemesis* (K92.0). Cough, selected by Rule 2, is ignored.

RULE B. *Trivial Conditions*

Where the selected cause is a trivial condition unlikely to cause death and a more serious condition is reported, reselect the underlying cause as if the trivial condition had not been reported. If the death was the result of an adverse reaction to treatment of the trivial condition, select the adverse reaction.

Example 3:

> I (a) Dental caries
> II   Cardiac arrest
>
> Code to *cardiac arrest* (I46.9) Dental caries, selected by the General Principle, is ignored.

Example 4:

> I (a) Ingrowing toenail and acute renal failure
>
> Code to *acute renal failure* (N17.9). Ingrowing toenail, selected by Rule 2, is ignored.

Example 5:

> I (a) Intraoperative haemorrhage
>   (b) Tonsillectomy
>   (c) Hypertrophy of tonsils
>
> Code to *haemorrhage during surgical operation* (Y60.0).

RULE C. *Linkage*

Where the selected cause is linked by a provision in the classification or in the notes for use in underlying cause mortality coding with one or more of the other conditions on the certificate, code the combination.

Example 6:

> I (a) Intestinal obstruction
>   (b) Femoral hernia
>
> Code to *femoral hernia with obstruction* (K41.3)

Example7:

> I (a) Right bundle-branch block and Chaga's disease

Code to *Chaga's disease with heart involvement* (B57.2). Right bundle-branch block, selected by Rule 2, links with Chaga's disease.

RULE D. *Specificity*

Where the selected cause describes a condition in general terms and a term that provides more precise information about the site or nature of this condition is reported on the certificate, prefer the more informative term.

Example 8:

> I (a) Cerebral infarction
>   (b) Cerebrovascular accident

Code to *cerebral infarction* (I63.9).

Example 9:

> I (a) Rheumatic heart disease, mitral stenosis

Code to *rheumatic mitral stenosis* (I05.0).

RULE E. *Early and late stages of disease*

Where the selected cause is an early stage of a disease and a more advanced stage of the same disease is reported on the certificate, code to the more advanced stage.

Example 10:

> I (a) Tertiary syphilis
>   (b) Primary syphilis

Code to *tertiary syphilis* (A52.9).

Example 11:

> I (a) Eclampsia during pregnancy
>   (b) Pre-eclampsia

Code to *eclampsia during pregnancy* (O15.0).

RULE F. *Sequelae*

Where the selected cause is an early form of a condition for which the classification provides a separate "Sequelae of \..." category, and there is evidence that death occurred from residual effects of this condition rather than from those of its active phase, code to the appropriate "Sequelae of ..." category.

Example 12:

        I (a) Pulmonary fibrosis
           (b) Old pulmonary tuberculosis

    Code to *sequelae of respiratory tuberculosis* (B90.9).

Example 13:

        I (a) Bronchopneumonia
          (b) Curvature of spine
          (c) Rickets in childhood

    Code to *sequelae of rickets* (E64.3).

Coding of Perinatal Mortality

You will notice that the perinatal mortality certificate has the following five sections for the entry of causes of perinatal deaths: -

    a) Main disease or condition in fetus or infant

    b) Other diseases or conditions in fetus or infant.

    c) Main maternal disease or condition affecting fetus or infant.

    d) Other maternal disease or condition affecting fetus or infant

    e) Other relevant circumstances

In section (a) and (b) should be entered diseases or conditions of the infant or fetus that made the greatest contribution to the death of the infant or fetus. In section (c) and (d) should be entered all diseases or conditions of the mother, that had some adverse effect on the infant or fetus. Section (e) is for the reporting of any other circumstance that may have a bearing on the death but cannot be described as a disease of the infant or mother, e.g. delivery in the absence of an attendant. The following example illustrates the statement of the causes of death for the case described:

A known diabetic, who was poorly controlled during her first pregnancy, developed megaloblastic anaemia at 32 weeks. There was also symptomless bacteriuria. Labour was induced at 38 weeks. There was spontaneous delivery of an infant weighing 3200g. The baby developed hypoglycaemia and died on the second day. Autopsy showed truncus arteriosus.

Causes of perinatal death:

a) Truncus arteriosus
b) Hypoglycaemia
c) Diabetes
d) Megaloblastic anaemia
e) Bacteriuria in pregnancy

On the Certificate of Cause of Perinatal Death this statement will be shown as follows:

CERTIFICATE OF CAUSE OF PERINATAL DEATH

To be completed for stillbirths and live born infants dying within 168 hours(1 week) from birth

Identifying particulars   ☐   This child was born live on   at   hours
                                                and died on   at   hours
                            ☐   This child was stillborn on   at   hours
                                and died before labour ☐ during labour ☐ not known ☐

Mother	Child
Date of birth ☐☐☐☐ 1st day of last ☐☐☐☐ menstrual period or, if known, age (years) ☐☐ or if unknown estimated duration of pregnancy ☐☐ (completed weeks) Number of previous pregnancies: Live births ☐☐ Still births ☐☐ Abortions ☐☐ Antenatal care, two or more visits: ☐ Yes ☐ No ☐ Not known Outcome of last previous pregnancy: ☐ Live birth Delivery: ☐ Stillbirth ☑ Normal spontaneous vertex ☐ Abortion other (specify) Date ☐☐☐	Birthweight: *3,200 grams* Sex: ☑ Boy ☐ Girl ☐ Indeterminate ☑Single birth ☐ First twin ☐Second twin ☐ Other multiple
	Attendant at birth
	☑ Physician ☐ Trained midwife Other trained person (specify) .... Other (specify) ....

Causes of death	
a. Main disease or condition in fetus or infant	*Truncus arteriosus*
b. Other diseases or conditions in fetus or infant	*Hypoglycaemia*
c. Main maternal disease or condition affecting fetus or infant	*Diabetes*
d. Other maternal diseases or conditions affecting fetus or infant	*Megaloblastic anaemia*
e. Other relevant circumstances	*Bacteriuria in pregnancy*

☐ The certified cause of death has been confirmed
   by autopsy
☐ Autopsy information may be available later
☐ Autopsy not being held

I certify.....................................
....
Signature and qualification

Before concluding this section on mortality, a word of caution. Make sure that you do not use certain codes in underlying cause mortality coding. These codes are listed in the following table:

TABLE 1. **Summary of codes not to be used in underlying cause mortality coding***

Codes not to be used for underlying cause mortality coding (code to item in parentheses; if no code is indicated, code to R99)		Not to be used if the underlying cause is known
B95-B97		F01-F09
E89.-		F70-F79
G97.-		G81.-
H59.-		G82.-
H95.-		G83.-
I15.-		H54.-
I23.-	(code to I21 or I22)	H90-H91
I24.0	(code to I21 or I22)	N46
I65.-	(code to I63)	N97.-
I66.-	(code to I63)	O30.-
I97.-		P07.-
J95.-		P08.-
K91.-		T79.-
M96.-		
N99.-		
O08.-		
O80.-O84	(code to O75.9)	
R69.-	(code to R95-R99)	
S00-T98	(code to V01-Y89)	
Y90-Y98		
Z00-Z99		

* *In addition to asterisk codes*

If all attempts to reach at the underlying cause of death fail or it is impossible to ascertain under what circumstances did the patient die, then code R99 ("unknown cause of mortality") or R98 ("found dead") can be used.

Details required for certifying cause of death

ICD-10 makes it possible to identify very precisely many varieties or sites of diseases and injuries and causal organisms. Although routine mortality statistics often list only broad classes of diseases, it is customary for the individual statistical record to store detailed information about the disease or injury. These records are valuable for research into particular conditions and for special statistical studies. Mortality statistics are much more meaningful if all details available in the deceased person's records regarding the precise diagnoses are incorporated in the death certificate.

The notes and examples which follow illustrate the method of completion of the international form of certification of causes of death and the degree of detail which can be stored using ICD-10. As a general rule, record diagnoses as precisely as information permits, incorporating relevant details from laboratory, histological or autopsy reports.

Infections

Acute, sub-acute or chronic; name of the disease and/or infecting organism, where known; the site, if localized; mode or transmission, where relevant; for syphilis, whether primary or secondary, congenital or acquired, early or late, clinical form, e.g.,

> Tuberculous meningitis
> Staphylococcal enterocolitis
> Bacillary dysentery due to Shigella boydii
> Mosquito-borne haemorrhagic fever
> Congenital syphilitic encephalitis
> Acute amoebic dysentery

Neoplasms

The morphological type, if known; malignant, benign, etc., if not specific to the morphology; site of origin of primary growths, stated as precisely as possible, and sites of secondary growths, clearly distinguished as such; if primary growth unknown or exact site within an organ not known, state accordingly; acute, subacute or chronic for leukaemias, e.g.,

Astrocytoma, temporal lobe, brain

Carcinoma, isthmus uteri

Carcinoma, endocervical canal

Malignant papilloma, bladder trigone

Hodgkin's paragranuloma

Chronic myeloid leukaemia

Endocrine disorders

Nature of disease process or disturbance of function; for thyroid disorders, whether toxic; for diabetes, state nature of complication or manifestation in a particular site, e.g.,

Panhypopituitarism

Corticoadrenal insufficiency

Diabetic nephropathy

Nutritional disorders

Type of deficiency, etc.; severity, where appropriate, e.g.,

Phenylketonuria

Pure hyperglyceridaemia

Blood disorders

Nature of disease process; type and nature of any deficiency of anaemia; whether hereditary, where relevant; nature of haemoglobinopathy; factor involved for coagulation defects, e.g.;

Pernicious anaemia
Scorbutic anaemia
Sickle-cell thalassaemia
Hereditary spherocytosis
Congenital Factor IX disorders

Nervous system disorders

Disease process; infecting organism, where relevant; whether hereditary, where relevant, e.g.,

Haemophilus influenzae meningoencephalits
Encephalitis due to mumps
Postvaccinal encephalomyelitis
Idiopathic Parkinson's disease
Hereditary peripheral neuropathy

Circulatory diseases

Nature of disease process; site, if localized; acute or chronic, where relevant; for rheumatic fever, whether active; specify rheumatic or other etiology for valvular heart conditions; any complications, e.g.,

Acute rheumatic pericarditis
Rheumatic mitral regurgitation
Hypertensive heart and renal disease
Coxsackie endocarditis
Thrombosis of basilar artery
Generalized atherosclerosis
Ruptured abdominal aortic aneurysm
Cerebral haemorrhage

Respiratory diseases

Nature of disease process; acute or chronic; infecting organism; any external cause, e.g.,

> Acute bronchitis
>
> Chronic obstructive bronchitis
>
> Pseudomonas pneumonia
>
> Aspergillosis
>
> Intrinsic asthma
>
> Pneumococcal serofibrinous pleurisy
>
> Idiopathic fibrosing alveolitis

Digestive diseases

Nature of disease process; site of ulcers, hernias, diverticula, etc,; acute ir chronic, where relevant; nature of any complication for ulcers, appendicitis, hernias, e.g.,

> Chronic duodenal ulcer with perforation
>
> Acute appendicitis with generalized peritonitis
>
> Gangrenous femoral hernia
>
> Crohn's disease of colon
>
> Diverticulosis of jejunum
>
> Pneumococcal peritonitis
>
> Alcoholic cirrhosis of liver
>
> Calculus of gallbladder with chronic cholecystitis
>
> Acute pancreatitis

Genitourinary disorders

Acute or chronic; clinical syndrome and pathological lesion for glomerulonephritis, etc,; site of calculi; infecting organism and site of infections; nature of complication, e.g.,

Nephrotic syndrome with lesion of membranoproliferative glomerulonephritis

Chronic glomerulonephritis with lesion of systemic lupus erythematosus

Chronic pyelonephritis

Acute renal failure with lesion of renal medullary necrosis

Hyperplasia of prostate

Gonococcal endometritis

Deaths associated with pregnancy, childbirth, and the puerperium

Nature of complication; whether obstruction occurred during labour; timing of death in relation to delivery; for abortions, whether spontaneous or induced; nature of complication; legal or illegal, if induced, e.g.,

Ruptured tubal pregnancy

Pelvic sepsis following illegally induced abortion

Amniotic fluid embolism following legally induced abortion

Severe pre-eclampsia; delivered by caesarean section

Obstructed labour due to transverse lie; delivery by breech extraction

Rupture of uterus during labour; delivery by forceps

Congenital anomalies

Site and type of anomaly; specify congenital if not obvious; complication, e.g.;

Spina bifida with hydrocephalus

Persistent ostium secundum

Congenital mitral stenosis

Congenital bronchiectasis

Atresia of colon

Perinatal deaths

Conditions in fetus or infant; conditions in mother or of placenta, cord or membranes. If believed to have affected the fetus or infant; for deaths from hypoxia or anoxia, state time of death in relation to onset of labour and to delivery; for deaths from birth asphyxia, state severity (or 1-minute Apgar score); for deaths associated with immaturity; state length of gestation and/or birthweight; whether light- or heavy-for-dates; type of birth trauma; infecting organism; whether transitory or permanent for endocrine or metabolic disturbances; cause of jaundice; type of blood grouping involved in iso-immunization (Rh, ABO, etc.); any complications, e.g.,

> Maternal tuberculosis
>
> Incompetent cervix
>
> Placenta praevia
>
> Light-for-dates with signs of fetal malnutrition
>
> Tentorial tear
>
> Fetal death from anoxia before onset of labour
>
> Severe birth asphyxia (1-minute Apgar score 2)
>
> Meconium pneumonitis
>
> Congenital toxoplasmosis
>
> Intrauterine Escherichia coli infection
>
> Kernicterus due to Rh isoimmunization
>
> Jaundice due to congenital obstruction of bile duct
>
> Neonatal thyrotoxicosis
>
> Idiopathic hydrops fetalis
>
> Extreme immaturity, birthweight 750 g

Injuries

Type of injury; site, stated as precisely as possible; complications, e.g.,

> Fracture of vault of skull
>
> Fracture of cervical vertebra with spinal cord lesion

Fracture of ileum

Open transcervical fracture of femur

Traumatic middle meningael haemorrhage

Rupture of kidney

Traumatic rupture of abdominal aorta

Poisoning

Substance involved; whether accidental, suicidal or homicidal.

Adverse effects of drugs in therapeutic use

State this fact; name of drug; nature of adverse effect; any complications; condition being treated, e.g.,

Aplastic anaemia due to therapeutic dosage of chloramphenicol
for urinary infection

Cushing's syndrome due to treatment with ACTH for severe rheumatoid
arthritis

Acute renal failure with renal papillary necrosis due to aspirin treatment
for arthritis

External cause of accidents

For transport accidents state vehicle involved; whether deceased was driver, passenger, etc., description of accident; place of occurrence; for other accidents specify circumstances and place of occurrence, e.g.

Passenger in car in collision with another car on the road

Accidental poisoning from carbon monoxide from car with engine
running in private garage

Fall from playground equipment on school premises

Burnt by flames from overturned stove in private house

Scorpion bite in the desert

Accidental drowning while playing in water

Struck by ball during game

Electrocuted by faulty electrical equipment at work

Suicide by hanging

Killed in fist fight

Examples of cause of death certification

Example 1

A man of 47 without previous history of coronary disease suffered a myocardial infarction and died 24 hours later.

It is sufficient to certify as follows:

I (a) Myocardial infarction — 1 day

      due to (or as a consequence of)

  (b) –

      due to (or as a consequence of)

  (c) –

II –

Example 2

A child of 18 months died of pneumonia following measles.

The direct cause of death is pneumonia and this can be considered to be "due to" the measles even if the pneumonia was a bacterial one.

I (a) Pneumonia — 6 days

      due to (or as a consequence of)

  (b) Measles — 3 weeks

      due to (or as a consequence of)

  (c) –

II –

The underlying cause is *measles*. Classification according to ICD-10 is to a subcategory of measles: *post-measles pneumonia*

Neoplasms

The morphological type, if known; malignant, benign, etc., if not specific to the morphology; site of origin of primary growths, stated as precisely as possible, and sites of secondary growths, clearly distinguished as such; if primary growth unknown or exact site within an organ not known, state accordingly; acute, sub-acute or chronic for leukaemias, e.g.,

Astrocytoma, temporal lobe, brain

Carcinoma, isthmus uteri

Carcinoma, endocervical canal

Malignant papilloma, bladder trigone

Hodgkin's paragranuloma

Chronic myeloid leukaemia

Endocrine disorders

Nature of disease process or disturbance of function; for thyroid disorders, whether toxic; for diabetes, state nature of complication or manifestation in a particular site, e.g.,

Panhypopituitarism

Corticoadrenal insufficiency

Diabetic nephropathy

Nutritional disorders

Type of deficiency, etc.; severity, where appropriate, e.g.,

Phenylketonuria

Pure hyperglyceridaemia

Blood disorders

Nature of disease process; type and nature of any deficiency of anaemia; whether hereditary, where relevant; nature of haemoglobinopathy; factor involved for coagulation defects, e.g.;

Example 5

A man of 49 died of a fracture of the vault of the skull, shortly after being involved in a collision between the car he was driving and a heavy truck on a narrow road.

I (a) Fracture of the vault of the skull –   15 minutes

     due to (or as a consequence of)

  (b) Collision between the car he was driving and heavy truck

     due to (or as a consequence of)

  (c) –

II –

Specify how and where the transport accident occurred. The underlying cause is the *collision between a motor vehicle and another motor vehicle on the highway*. The deceased person is specified as the driver.

Example 6

A woman of 74 suffering from residual hemipraesis following a celebral thrombosis several years ago fell at home and fractured the neck of her femur. During immobilization following the injury, she developed hypostatic pneumonia, from which she died.

I (a) Hypostatic pneumonia   –   1 day

     due to (or as a consequence of)

  (b) Immobilization   –   2 months

     due to (or as a consequence of)

  (c) Pertrochanteric fracture of femur   –   2 months

     due to (or as a consequence of)

  (d) Tripped and fell at home   –   2 months

II Hemipraesis from old celebral thrombosis–   5 years

The hemipraesis may have contributed to the fall but is not considered to be part of the direct sequence of cause leading to death. Specify how the fall occurred and the site of fracture. The underlying cause is *"fall on same level from slipping, tripping or stumbling."*

Example 7

A woman of 48 died of shock following removal of gallbladder for acute cholecystitis arising from gallstones, chronic glomerulonephritis also being present.

I (a) Postoperative shock

      due to (or as a consequence of)

  (b) Cholecystectomy for acute cholecystitis

      due to (or as a consequence of)

  (c) Cholelithiasis

II Chronic membranoproliferative glomerulonephritis

Specify acute or chronic cholecystitis and indicate site of calculi. The underlying cause is <u>cholelithiasis</u>. ICD-10 allows classification to "calculus of gallbladder with acute cholecystitis". Specify acute of chronic and pathological lesion in glomerulonephritis.

Example 8

A man of 63 had been treated for some years for malignant hypertension and developed hypertensive heart disease and chronic renal failure. While seriously ill with heart condition, he developed acute appendicitis and appendix ruptured. Appendicectomy was carried out successfully, but the heart condition deteriorated further and he died 2 weeks later.

I (a) Congestive heart failure

      due to (or as a consequence of)

  (b) Cardiac hypertrophy

      due to (or as a consequence of)

  (c) Malignant hypertension

II Appendicectomy for acute appendicitis with rupture of appendix. Hypertensive renal failure,

The appendicitis and operation are thought to have accelerated the original condition but they were not part of the fatal sequence. In generalized conditions such as hypertension or arteriosclerosis, state organ mainly involved in the events leading to death. Indicate clearly the link between the hypertension and renal conditions in Part II. Specify complications of appendicitis. The underlying cause is <u>malignant hypertension</u>. ICD-10 allows classification to <u>malignant hypertensive heart disease</u>.

Example 9

A woman of 48 with secondary carcinoma of the vertebral column died of bronchopneumonia. Extensive investigations had failed to reveal the site of the primary growth.

I (a) Bronchopneumonia   –   1 week

      due to (or as a consequence of)

  (b) Secondary carcinoma of vertebral column (primary site unknown) – 3 years

      due to (or as a consequence of)

  (c) –

The long illness was considered to have paved the way for the development of the bronchopneumonia.. The underlying cause is <u>malignant neoplasm of unknown site</u>.

Example 10

A man of 87 with clinically diagnosed carcinoma of stomach, never operated on, died of generalized carcinomatosis.

I (a) Carcinomatosis   –   1 month

      due to (or as a consequence of)

  (b) Carcinoma of stomach (part unknown) –   1 year

Give the fullest details known about the site of neoplasms or state if the exact location is unknown. It is likely that the statistical office will inquire for further details if the site is not specified so as to allow classification as precisely as the ICD permits.

Example 11

A woman of 38 died of cardiac arrest shortly after a caesarean operation had been carried out because of obstruction during labour caused by locked twins. Attempts at resuscitation were unsuccessful.

I (a) Cardiac arrest–   Instantaneous

    due to (or as a consequence of)

  (b) Caesarean section   –   1/2 hour ·

    due to (or as a consequence of)

  (c) Locked twins causing obstruction in labor   –   4 hours

The specified cause is *obstructed labour due to locked twins.*

Example 12

The following illustrates the importance of accurately stating the sequence of morbid conditions in order to allow selection of the cause considered "underlying" by the attending physician. A diabetic man who had been under insulin control for many years developed ischaemic heart disease and died suddenly from a myocardial infarction. Most people consider there to be a relationship between diabetes and ischaemic heart disease but its nature is not yet fully understood. Depending on the role the doctor considers to have played in the fatal outcome by one or the other conditions, the following certifications are possible:

1. If the doctor considered that the heart condition resulted from the long-standing diabetes, the sequence would be:

I (a) Myocardial infarction   –   1 hour

    due to (or as a consequence of)

(b) Chronic ischaemic heart disease –   5 years

     due to (or as a consequence of)

(c) Diabetes mellitus   –   12 years

and the statistical office would select *diabetes* as the underlying cause of death.

2. If the doctor considered that the heart condition developed independently of the diabetes, the certification would be:

I (a) Myocardial infarction   –   1 hour

     due to (or as a consequence of)

   (b) Chronic ischaemic heart disease –   5 years

II.   Diabetes mellitus   –   12 years

And the *heart condition* would be recorded as the underlying cause.

3. If the man had instead died from some other complications of the diabetes, such as nephropathy, the heart condition playing only a subsidiary part in the death and the doctor being uncertain that it arose from the diabetes at all, the certificate should be in the form:

I (a) Acute renal failure   –   1 week

     due to (or as a consequence of)

   (b) Nephropathy –   4 years

     due to (or as a consequence of)

   (c) Diabetes mellitus   –   12 years

II.   Chronic ischaemic heart disease–   5 years

The underlying cause is *diabetic nephropathy*.

Each of the above certifications would be accepted by the statistical office as it stands. Sometimes, however, certificates are received in this form:

I (a) Diabetes mellitus

     due to (or as a consequence of)

(b) Myocardial infarction

This is an impossible sequence since I (a) could not be "due to" I (b); it indicates that the certifier did not understand the way the certificate is intended to be used. In such a case, the safest course is for the statistical office to enquire from the certifier what he/she really meant to say.

PERINATAL DEATHS

In the preceding examples we have been following the principle of a single underlying cause for tabulation of mortality in general. Experience has shown that it is less useful in perinatal mortality where two separate individuals, i.e. mother and baby, are involved and when causes or circumstances not necessarily attributable to mother and child could contribute to the event of perinatal death.

To accommodate such conditions, a separate form has been recommended by the W.H.O. for the certification of perinatal mortality which has been reproduced earlier. Some examples are given below to make the concept clearer and to suggest the proper way of certifying perinatal mortality.

Example 1

A 26 year old woman had a normal pregnancy and delivered a baby at full term. The newborn however was found dead at delivery. It was difficult to arrive at a definite cause of death with performing an autopsy.

Causes of perinatal death:

a) Fetal death, cause unknown

b) –

c) –

d) –

e) –

Example 2

A woman, 32 years old, delivered a stillborn child at 38 weeks. The infant weighed 750g and showed signs of antepartum anoxia and fetal malnutrition. The mother suffered from placenta praevia and toxaemia during the latter half of her pregnancy.

Causes of perinatal death:

    a) Fetal malnutrition

    b) Antepartum anoxia

    c) Toxaemia

    d) Placenta praevia

    e) Bacteriuria in pregnancy

Example 3

The patient was a 30 year old woman with a healthy 4 year old boy. There was a normal pregnancy apart from hydramnios. X-ray at 36 weeks suggested anencephaly. Labour was induced. A stillborn anencephalic fetus was delivered.

Causes of perinatal death:

    a) Anencephaly

    b) –

    c) Hydramnios

    d) –

    e) –

Example 4

A primigravida, 19, who had been severely pre-eclamptic at the end of her pregnancy, suffered through long period of obstructed labour. She delivered a hydrocephalic boy who died 30 minutes later due to asphyxia sustained during birth.

Causes of perinatal death:

    a) Congenital hydrocephalus

    b) Severe birth asphyxia

c) Obstructed labour

d) Severe pre-eclampsia

Example 5

A 32 year old multiparous mother, suffering from chronic glomerulonephritis, underwent forceps delivery and gave birth to a liveborn child who died of umbilical haemorrhage 30 minutes after birth.

Causes of perinatal death:

   a) Umbilical haemorrhage after birth

   b) –

   c) Chronic glomerulonephritis

   d) Forceps delivery

   e) Maternal pre-eclampsia, mild

Example 6

A 20 year old primigravida, after having prolonged labour delivered a liveborn baby boy. Forceps were used during delivery and the baby sustained scalp injuries in the process. Neonatal haemorrhage was also recorded. The child died 2 days after birth.

Causes of perinatal death:

   a) Injuries to scalp

   b) Neonatal haemorrhage

   c) Forceps delivery

   d) Prolonged labour

Exercise 8

1. From the list of choices given below, select the one (by encircling it) that completes the sentence. The *underlying cause of death* is the condition, event or circumstance:

   a) Which was the immediate or direct cause of death.
   b) Without which the patient would not have died.
   c) Which originally resulted in admission to hospital.
   d) Which gave the patient the greatest suffering.

2. Which do you think is the underlying cause of death (by encircling your choice) in the following diagnosis?

   Coma from brain hemorrhage after falling from balcony
   a) Coma
   b) Brain hemorrhage
   c) Fall from balcony

3. Fill in the blanks to complete the following sentences:

   a) The responsibility for deciding on the logical sequence of deaths lies with the certifying ....

   b) In case of deaths due to injury, it is the .... code (Chapter ....) that should be used for single cause coding and tabulating underlying cause.

   c) The .... code should not be used for mortality coding. The dagger code is the .... code for this purpose.

   d) According to the General Principle when more than one condition is entered on the certificate, the condition entered on the .... used line of part .... should be selected .... if it could have given rise to .... the conditions entered .... it.

UNIT 9
PRESENTATION OF STATISTICS

UNIT 9
PRESENTATION OF STATISTICS

Introduction

Health care statistics are usually used for two main reasons: for the management of national healthcare delivery system, and for international comparison. Both require consistency and standardization. To this end, WHO has formulated a set of guidelines for data presentation in national statistics, and regulations regarding statistics for international comparison. It has also laid down standard definitions related to morbidity and mortality, specified numerators and denominators for ratios and rates, and made recommendations in relation to statistical tables for international comparison. The users of ICD-10 and health statisticians are well advised to make themselves familiar with such guidelines, recommendations and definitions. This would not only render greater credibility to health related statistics of a particular nation but also greater confidence in presenting its statistics for international comparison.

WHO definitions

1. **Live birth**

   Live birth is the complete expulsion from its mother, of the fetus, irrespective of the duration of pregnancy, which breathes or shows any other evidence of life (e.g. beating of the heart, pulsation of the umbilical cord, or definite movement of voluntary muscles).

2. **Fetal death**

   Fetal death is death prior to the complete expulsion, from its mother, of the fetus, irrespective of the duration of pregnancy. The death is indicated by the fact that after such separation the fetus does not breathe or show any other evidence of life (e.g. beating of the heart, pulsation of the umbilical cord, or definite movement of voluntary muscles.

3. Birth weight

It is the first weight of the fetus or newborn obtained after birth. It should be measured within the first hour of life before significant postnatal weight loss has occurred. The average weight of the newborn is approximately 7 pounds or 3,200 grams.

   i)   Low birth weight (less than 2500g)
   ii)   Very low birth weight (less than 1500g)
   iii)   Extremely low birth weight (less than 1000g)

4. Gestational age

The duration of gestation is measured from the first day of the last normal menstrual period. Gestational age is expressed in completed days or completed weeks (e.g. events occurring 280 to 286 completed days after the onset of the last normal menstrual period are considered to have occurred at 40 weeks of gestation).

5. Pre-term

Less than 37 completed weeks (less than 259 days) of gestation.

6. Term

From 37 completed weeks to less than 42 completed weeks (259 to 293 days) of gestation.

7. Post-term

42 completed weeks or more (294 days or more) of gestation.

8. Perinatal period

The perinatal period commences at 22 completed weeks (154 days) of gestation (the time when birth weight is normally 500g), and ends seven completed days after birth.

9. Neonatal period

The neonatal period commences at birth and ends 28 completed days after birth. Neonatal deaths (deaths among live births during the first 28 completed days of life may be subdivided into *early neonatal deaths*, occurring during the *first seven days* of life, and *late neonatal deaths*, occurring after the seventh day but before 28 completed days of life.

10. Maternal death

A maternal death is the death of a woman while pregnant or within 42 days of termination of pregnancy, irrespective of the duration and the site of the pregnancy, from any cause related to or aggravated by the pregnancy or its management, but not from accidental or incidental **causes.**

11. Late maternal death

A late maternal death is the death of a woman from direct or indirect obstetric causes more than 42 days but less than one year after termination of pregnancy.

12. Pregnancy-related death

A pregnancy-related death is the death of a woman while pregnant or within 42 days of termination of pregnancy, irrespective of the cause of death.

Maternal deaths should be divided into two groups:

Direct obstetric deaths: those resulting from obstetric complications of the pregnant state (pregnancy, labour and puerperium) from interventions, omissions, incorrect treatment, or from a chain of events resulting from any of the above.

Indirect obstetric deaths: those resulting from previous existing disease or disease that developed during pregnancy and which was not due to direct obstetric causes, but which was aggravated by physiologic effects of pregnancy.

Ratios and rates

Care must be observed in specifying numerators and denominators (i.e. live births, total births, or live births plus fetal deaths) in calculating mortality. As per WHO requirements results should be expressed as a ratio of the numerator to the denominator, multiplied by 'k', which may be 1000, 10,000 or 100,000, as preferred and indicated by the country.

a) Fetal death ratio

$$\frac{\text{Fetal deaths}}{\text{Live births}} \times 1000$$

b) Fetal death rate

$$\frac{\text{Fetal deaths}}{\text{Total births}} \times 1000$$

c) Fetal death rate, weight-specific

$$\frac{\text{Fetal deaths weighing 1000g and over}}{\text{Total births weighing 1000g and over}} \times 1000$$

d) Early neonatal mortality rate

$$\frac{\text{Early neonatal deaths}}{\text{Live births}} \times 1000$$

e) Early neonatal mortality rate, weight specific

$$\frac{\text{Early neonatal deaths of infants weighing 1000g and over at birth}}{\text{Live births weighing 1000g and over}} \times 1000$$

f) Perinatal mortality ratio

$$\frac{\text{Fetal deaths and early neonatal deaths}}{\text{Live births}} \times 1000$$

g) Perinatal mortality rate

$$\frac{\text{Fetal deaths and early neonatal deaths}}{\text{Total births}} \times 1000$$

h) Perinatal mortality rate, weight-specific

$$\frac{\text{Fetal deaths weighing 1000g and over, plus early neonatal deaths of infants weighing 1000g and over at birth}}{\text{Total births weighing 1000g and over}} \times 1000$$

i) Neonatal mortality rate

$$\frac{\text{Neonatal deaths}}{\text{Live births}} \times 1000$$

j) Neonatal mortality rate, weight-specific

$$\frac{\text{Neonatal deaths of infants weighing 1000g and over at birth}}{\text{Live births weighing 1000g and over}} \times 1000$$

k) Infant mortality rate

$$\frac{\text{Deaths under one year of age}}{\text{Live births}} \times 1000$$

l) Infant mortality rate, weight-specific

$$\frac{\text{Infant deaths among live births weighing 1000g and over at birth}}{\text{Live births weighing 1000g and over}} \times 1000$$

m) Maternal mortality rate

$$\frac{\text{Maternal deaths (direct and indirect)}}{\text{Live births}} \times k$$

n) Direct obstetric mortality ratio

$$\frac{\text{Direct obstetric deaths only}}{\text{Live births}} \times k$$

o) **Pregnancy-related mortality ratio**

$$\frac{\text{Pregnancy-related deaths}}{\text{Live births}} \quad X \quad k$$

Special tabulation lists as recommended by the WHO

Because the full four-character list of the ICD, and even the three-character list, is too long to be presented in every statistical table, most routine statistics use a tabulation list that emphasizes certain single conditions and group others. The four special lists for the tabulation of mortality are an integral part of the ICD. Lists 1 and 2 are for general mortality and lists 3 and 4 are for infant and child mortality (ages 0 to 4 years). There is also a special tabulation list for morbidity.

The special tabulation lists for mortality

The special tabulation lists for mortality are given in Volume 1. These are of two types:

a) **The condensed list**

The two condensed lists, List 1 and List 3, provide items for each ICD chapter and also, within most chapters, identify the items of the selected lists together with residual items entitled "Remainder of ...", which complete the coverage of the respective chapter. They thus condense the full range of ICD three-character categories into a manageable number of items for many publication purposes.

b) **The selected lists**

The two selected lists, List 2 and List 4, contain items within most ICD chapters, for conditions and external causes significant for the monitoring and analysis of population health status and mortality-related health concerns at both national and international levels. Chapter totals are not provided and only a few chapters have residual categories that enable such totals to be obtained.

The special tabulation list for morbidity

The tabulation list for morbidity contains 298 detailed items. The morbidity list is a condensed list in which each category is included only once and totals for groups of diseases and ICD chapters can be obtained by the addition of sequential items.

The morbidity lists is intended as a basis for national list and for inter-country comparison. National lists can be constructed by either condensing or expanding the core classification as appropriate. The list is suitable for data on inpatient care and, with suitable adaptation – notably aggregation of some items and expansion of items relating to Chapter XVIII (symptoms, signs and abnormal clinical and laboratory findings) and Chapter XXI (factors influencing health status and contact with health services) – for information from other sources such as outpatient care and health surveys.

Modification of the special tabulation lists for local use

a) Mortality lists

The four special tabulation lists provide for most countries an adequate source of information about the most important diseases and external causes of death. They also facilitate comparison over time and observation of shifts in the relative frequencies of, for example, infectious diseases and degenerative diseases, as health programmes take effect. They make possible meaningful international comparisons of causes of death.

When there is no need for international comparison, lists similar to the special tabulation lists can be designed for use locally. The ICD categories of such lists can be selected and grouped in whatever way is most appropriate and useful.

b) Morbidity lists

The special tabulation list for morbidity can also be modified according to local or national requirements. If after the examination of the frequencies of the ICD three-character categories, it is felt necessary to expand the list, some of the items for a range of ICD categories can be subdivided according to the core classification or even to the four-character level. If the recommended list is required, selection could be made based on national or local health concerns. Depending on a country's morbidity status, categories may be combined to shorten the list.

Statistical tables

WHO has made specific recommendations in relation to statistical tables for international comparison. The following patterns, which are designed to promote international, comparability, present standard ways of expressing various characteristics such as cause, sex, age and geographical area.

(a) Analysis by the International Classification of Diseases should, as appropriate, be in accordance with:

    (i)   the detailed list of three-character categories, with or without four-character subcategories;

    (ii)   one of the special tabulation lists for mortality;

    (iii) the special tabulation list for morbidity.

(b) Age classification for general purposes:

    (i)   under 1 year, single years to 4 years, 5-year groups from 5 to 84 years, 85 years and over;

    (ii)   under 1 year, 1-4 years, 5-14 years, 15-24 years, 25-34 years, 35-44 years, 45-54 years, 55-64 years, 65-74 years, 75 years and over.

    (iii)   Under 1 year, 1-4 years, 15-44 years, 45-64 years, 65 years and over.

(c) Classification by area should, as appropriate, be in accordance with:

    (i)   each major civil division;

    (ii)   each town or conurbation of 1,000,000 population and over, otherwise the largest town with a population of at least 100,000;

    (iii)   a national aggregate of urban areas of 100,000 population and over;

    (iv)   a national aggregate of urban areas of less than 100,000 population;

    (v)   a national aggregate of rural areas.

Tabulation of causes of death

1. Statistics of causes of death for a defined area should be in accordance with recommendation (a) (i) above, or, if this is not possible, with recommendation (a) (ii). Deaths should preferably be classified by sex and age group as in recommendation (b) (i).

2. Statistics of causes of deaths for the areas in recommendation (c) should comply with recommendation (a) (ii), or if this is not possible, with recommendation (a) (iii). They should preferably be tabulated by sex and age group as in recommendation (b) (ii).

3. In countries where medical certification of the cause of death is incomplete or limited to certain areas, figures for deaths not medically certified should be published separately.

4. The legal requirements for the registration of fetal deaths and live births vary from country to country. If possible, all fetuses and infants weighing at least 500g at birth, whether alive or dead, should be included in the statistics.

5. When information on birth weight is unavailable, the corresponding criteria for gestational age (22 completed weeks) or body length (25 on crown-heel) should be used.

6. The criteria for deciding whether an event has taken place within the perinatal period should be applied in the order: 1) birth weight, 2) gestational age, 3) crown-heel length.

Presentation of causes of perinatal mortality

For statistics of perinatal mortality derived from the form or certificate recommended for this purpose (see unit 8), full-scale multiple-cause analysis of all conditions reported will be desirable. Where it is not possible, analysis of the main disease or condition in the fetus or infant (part a) and of the main maternal condition affecting the fetus or infant (part c) with cross tabulation of groups of these two conditions should be regarded as the minimum. When it is necessary to select only one condition, the main disease or condition in the fetus or infant (part a) should be selected.

Age classification for special statistics of infant mortality

(i) By single days for the first week of life (under 24 hours, 1, 2, 3, 4, 5, 6 days), 7-13 days, 14-20 days, 21-27 days, 28 days and up to, but not including, 2 months, by single months of life from 2 months to 1 year (2, 3, 4 ....11 months).

(ii)   Under 24 hours, 1-6 days, 7-27 days, 28 days up to, but not including, 3 months, 3-5 months, 6 months but under 1 year.

(iii)   Under 7 days, 7-27 days, 28 days but less than 1 year.

Age classification for early neonatal deaths

(i)   Under 1 hour, 1-11 hours, 12-23 hours, 24-47 hours, 48-71 hours, 72-167 hours;

(ii)   Under 1 hour, 1-23 hours, 24-167 hours.

Birth weight classification for perinatal mortality statistics

By weight intervals of 500 g, i.e. 1000-1499 g, etc.

Gestational age classification for perinatal mortality statistics

Under 28 weeks (under 196 days), 28-31 weeks (196-223 days), 32-36 weeks (224-258 days), 37-41 weeks (259-293 days), 42 weeks and over (294 days and over).

Whatever list of causes is being used, it may be found that no cases occur in certain cells of a statistical table. Where there are many empty lines in a table, it is advisable to omit such lines from a published table or from a computer printout. When only the occasional case of a disease occurs in a country, the line can be regularly omitted from the published table and a footnote added to indicate either that there were no cases or, when sporadic cases do occur, in which cell the case would have appeared.

UNIT 10
APPENDICES
(A – C)

APPENDIX A

LIST OF WHO COLLABORATING CENTRES FOR CLASSIFICATION OF DISEASES

Ten WHO Collaboration Centres for the Family of International Classifications have been established to assist countries with problems encountered in the development and use of health-related classifications and, in particular, in the use of ICD.

There are three centres for English-language users. Communications may be addressed to the Head, WHO Collaborating Centre for Classification of Diseases at:

1. Australian Institute of Health
   GPO Box 570
   Canberra ACT 2601
   Australia.

2. Office for National Statistics
   1 Drummond Gate
   London, SW1V 2QQ
   England.

3. National Centre for Health Statistics
   Centre for Disease Control and Prevention
   3311 Toledo Road
   Hyattsville, MD 20782
   U.S.A.

The other seven centres, each based on an individual language or group of languages, are located in the following institutions:

1. Peking Union Medical College Hospital
   Chinese Academy of Medical Sciences
   Beijing 100730

China (for Chinese)

2. INSERM

   44 Chemin de Ronde

   F - 78110 Le Vesinet

   France (for French)

3. Department of Social Medicine

   University Hospital

   S – 751 85 Uppsala

   Sweden (for the Nordic Countries)

4. Faculdade de Saude Publica

   Universidade de Sao Paulo

   Avenida Dr Arnaldo 715

   0255 Sao Panlo, SP

   Brazil (for Portuguese)

5. The N.A. Semasko Institute

   U 1. Obuha 12

   Moscow B - 120

   Russian Federation (for Russian)

6. German Institute of Medical Information

   Waisenhausgasse 36-38 A

   50676 Koln

   Germany (for German)

7. Centro Venezolano de Classification de Enfermedades

   El Silencio

   Centro Simon Bolivar

   Edificio Sir, Piso 3, Oficina 315

   Caracas 1010

   Venezuela (for Spanish)

APPENDIX B: ICD-9 and ICD-10: A COMPARATIVE LOOK

Main Changes

In this section we shall consider how ICD-10 has changed from ICD-9 in its basic design. The changes are significant but, if you are familiar with ICD-9, they should not cause you any major problems.

The three main changes are:

1. There are now three volumes in ICD-10.
2. There are now 22 chapters.
3. The structure of the code has changed.

We shall now look at each of these changes in detail.

1. The three volumes of ICD-10 have been created by splitting:

Vol. 1 of ICD-9 into   ⟶   Vol. 1, and

                     ⟶   Vol. 2 in ICD-10

Vol. 2 of ICD-9 becomes ⟶ Vol. 3 in ICD-10, with

                                   little change in structure

2. The major structural change in ICD-10 is that there are 22 chapters in it as compared to the 17 chapters of ICD-9. In fact there have been 17 chapters since ICD-9 was introduced in 1929!

The additional 4 chapters in ICD-10 have arisen as follows:

ICD-9 Chapter VI (Diseases of the Nervous System and Sense Organs) has been split into 3 chapters in ICD-10, namely.

         Chapter VI   - Diseases of the nervous system

         Chapter VII   - Diseases of the eye and adnexa

         Chapter VIII - Diseases of the ear and mastoid process.

And, by bringing the two supplementary classifications -- the E and V codes -- into the main part of the ICD.

Thus, the 'E' codes become

Chapter XX – External causes of morbidity & mortality and

The V codes become

Chapter XXI – Factors influencing health status and contact with health services.

3. The third significant change in ICD-10 is the structure of the code. The first character of the code is now an alphabetical character.

In ICD-10 the category code is made up of one alphabetic and two numeric characters as opposed to three numeric characters in ICD-9.

For example: Code 375 in ICD-9 becomes H04 in ICD-10. Note that the use of an alphabetical character at the beginning of the code has increased the number of available three-character codes to 2600 instead of the 1000 in ICD-9. This in turn vastly increases the number of four-character sub-categories available (approximately 60% more).

Other Changes

In brief, what you would find as new in ICD-10 is highlighted as follows:

a) Replacement of the traditional numeric coding system with an alphanumeric scheme with the aim of stabilizing the coding system and minimizing disruptions at future revisions.

b) Greatly expanded explanatory notes and instructions for use.

c) Considerable expansion of the dagger and asterisk system of dual classification, with the asterisk information contained in homogenous categories at the 3-character level.

d) New chapters for diseases of the eye and adnexa, and diseases of the ear and mastoid process.

e) Revised definitions, standards, and reporting requirements for maternal, fetal, perinatal, neonatal, and infant mortality.

f) New categories for coding post-procedural disorders.

g) Greater coding precision for drug-induced conditions.

The following table lists the important differences between ICD-9 and ICD-10 in greater details.

ICD-9	ICD-10
1. Introduced in 1977.	1. Introduced in 1994.
2. Entitled "International Classification of Diseases, Injuries, and Causes of Death.	2. Entitled "International Statistical Classification of Diseases and Related Health Problems.
3. Brought out in 2 volumes: (Vol. 1. Tabular List) (Vol. 2. Alphabetical Index)	3. Brought out in 3 Volumes. (Vol. 1: Tabular List) (Vol. 2: Instruction Manual) (Vol. 3: Alphabetical Index)
4. Totally numeric in nature.	4. Alpha-numeric in nature
5. Has 17 main chapters and 2 special, supplementary chapters.	5. Has 22 chapters and no supplementary chapters.
6. Has an "E" & "V" supplementary classifications.	6. "E" & "V" Supplementary Classifications incorporated as parts of the core classification.
7. Includes the "Basic Tabulation List".	7. "Basic Tabulation List" withdrawn.

ICD-9	ICD-10
8. Two short lists (each of 50 causes) introduced to list morbidity & mortality.	8. These short lists withdrawn and replaced by 5 newly designed lists.
9. A separate classification, termed "Classification of Industrial Accidents, According to Injury" introduced.	9. This Classification scheme withdrawn altogether.
10. "Medical Certification & Rules for Classification" component as part of Volume1, the *Tabulation List*.	10. This component removed from Volume1 and features, in greatly revised form, in Vol. 2, the *Instruction Manual*.
11. Cause of Death component of the standard WHO Death Certificate has 3 lines (a, b, & c).	11. An additional line (line'd') has been introduced to bring greater accuracy in determining the precise underlying cause of death.
12. Provided no guidelines about presenting statistical data in a standard format.	12. Has a special chapter in Vol.2 ("Statistical Presentation") for this purpose.
13. Alternative forms of diseases or conditions indicated by indenting them under the main condition.	13. Use of "bullets" (.) to indicate alternative forms of a disease or condition.
14. "Diseases of the Nervous System & Sense Organs" presented in Chapter VI.	14. Chapter VI has been split into 3 chapters (Diseases of the nervous system, Diseases of eye & adnexa, and Diseases of the ear & mastoid process).
15. No provision for *Post-procedural* Disorders which often constitute a medical care problem right.	15. New categories are created at the end of certain chapters for *Postprocedural Disorders*.

ICD-9	ICD-10
16. Provided separate "Late Effects" category for each intent (i.e. suicide, accident, homicide, etc.) for an injury.	16. All such categories have been brought together in a block entitled "external causes of morbidity & mortality".
17. "Type of Injury" was used as the axis of classification and then sub-classified the type of injury according to the "Site of Injury".	17. Injuries are coded first to the "Body Region" where the injury has occurred, then to the "Type of Injury".
18. The main axis of classification for land transport accidents was whether the event was a traffic or non-traffic accident.	18. The main axis for this type of accident is now the injured person's "mode of transport".
19. "Corrosion" and "burns" were coded to the same set of codes as all other types of burns.	19. Each 3-character category in the block identifies "Corrosions" and "Burns" separately at the 4-character level.
20. "Friction Burns" were classified with "Superficial Injuries".	20. "Friction burns" are included with "Burns".
21. No "Activity code" existed in the chapter for External Causes of Injury & Poisoning".	21. An "Activity code" is provided in Chapter XX (External Causes of Injury & Poisoning) for optional use to indicate the activity of the person at the time of the accident.
22. Both, the "lead term" and "modifiers" in vol.2 (Index) were printed in usual normal size letters.	22. The "lead terms" in vol.3 (Index) are printed in bold letters to improve the readability of the Index.
23. No provision for updating the ICD between Revisions -- such activity possible after every ten years.	23. Provision for updating ICD between Revisions by issuing a small number of amendments annually.

EXERCISE 9

Identify and list the three main changes in ICD-10 as compared
to ICD-9

1. ....

2. ....

3. ....

APPENDIX C

THE WHO FAMILY OF INTERNATIONAL CLASSIFICATIONS

The WHO family of International Classifications (WHO-FIC) attempts to serve as the framework of international standards to provide the building blocks of health information systems. The following is a schematic representation of the WHO-FIC.

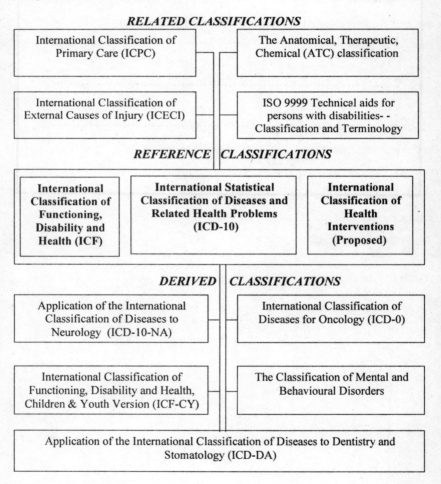

RELATED CLASSIFICATIONS

International Classification of Primary Care (ICPC)	The Anatomical, Therapeutic, Chemical (ATC) classification
International Classification of External Causes of Injury (ICECI)	ISO 9999 Technical aids for persons with disabilities- - Classification and Terminology

REFERENCE CLASSIFICATIONS

International Classification of Functioning, Disability and Health (ICF)	International Statistical Classification of Diseases and Related Health Problems (ICD-10)	International Classification of Health Interventions (Proposed)

DERIVED CLASSIFICATIONS

Application of the International Classification of Diseases to Neurology (ICD-10-NA)	International Classification of Diseases for Oncology (ICD-0)
International Classification of Functioning, Disability and Health, Children & Youth Version (ICF-CY)	The Classification of Mental and Behavioural Disorders

Application of the International Classification of Diseases to Dentistry and Stomatology (ICD-DA)

Reference Classifications

These are the classifications that cover the main parameters of the health system, such as death, disease, functioning, disability, health and health interventions. WHO reference classifications are a product of international agreements. They have achieved broad acceptance and official agreement for use and are approved and recommended as guidelines for international reporting on health. They may be used as models for the development or revision of other classifications with respect to both the structure and the character and definition of the classes.

Currently there are two reference classifications in the WHO-FIC: ICD as a reference classification to capture information on mortality and morbidity and ICF to capture information on various domains of human functioning and disability. WHO has been exploring to the possibility of replacing the former International Classification of Procedures in Medicine by a new International Classification of Health Interventions (ICHI).

Derived Classifications

Derived classifications are based upon reference classifications. Derived classifications may be prepared either by adopting the reference classification structure and classes, providing additional detail beyond that provided by the reference classification or they may be prepared through rearrangement or aggregation of items from one or more reference classifications. Derived classifications are often tailored for use at the national or international level.

Within the WHO-FIC the derived classifications include specialty-based adaptations of ICF and ICD, such as the International Classification of Diseases for Oncology (ICD-0), the Application of the International Classification of Diseases to Dentistry and Stomatology (ICD-DA), the ICD-10 for Mental and Behavioural Disorders and the Application of the International Classification of Diseases to Neurology (ICD-10-NA).

Related Classifications

Related classifications are those that partially refer to reference classifications, or that are associated with the reference classifications at specific levels of the structure only. Procedures for maintaining, updating and revising statistical classifications of the family encourage the resolution of problems of partial correspondence among related classifications, and offer opportunities for increased harmony over time. Within the WHO-FIC the related classifications include: the International Classification of Primary Care (ICPC-2), the International Classification of External Causes of Injury (ICECI), Technical aids for persons with disabilities: Classification and terminology (ISO9999) and the Anatomical, Therapeutic, Chemical Classification (ATC).

KEY TO ANSWERS

UNIT EXERCISES
(1-9)

Exercise 1

1. ICD is an abbreviation for International *Classification* of *Diseases*.
2. The initials WHO stand for *World Health Organization*.
3. Diagnostic coding is used to assist record retrieval and produce *statistics*.
4. The two main reasons, for which mortality & morbidity statistics are collected, are: *Epidemiology* and *Medical care management*.
5. *Epidemiology* is the study of the distribution and determinates of disease frequency.
6. The three epidemiological characteristics of the newborn on which it is important to collect statistics, are:
   > *Birth weight*
   > *Length of gestation*
   > *Type of delivery*
7. A classification is an orderly *arrangement* of objects or individuals into *groups* on the basis of certain characteristics.

Exercise 2

1. F	3. T	5. T	7. F	9. F
2. F	4. T	6. F	8. T	10. T

Exercise 3.1

CHAPTER	MARK	CHAPTER	MARK
" I	S	" XII	B
" II	S	" XIII	B
" III	S	" XIV	B
" IV	S	" XV	S
" V	S	" XVI	S
" VI	B	" XVII	S
" VII	B	" XVIII	G
" VIII	B	" XIX	S
" IX	B	" XX	E
" X	B	" XXI	E
" XI	B	" XXII	S

Exercise 3.2

1. B   3. S   5. S
2. B   4. B   6. S

Exercise 3.3

a) Diseases generally recognized as communicable or transmissible.
b) Influenza and other acute respiratory infections.
c) In categories J00 to J22.
d) Yes, category A06 (Amoebiasis) includes both terms

Exercise 3.4

1. Profound mental retardation.
2. "IQ under 20 (in adults, mental age below 3 years). Results in severe limitation in self-care, continence, communication and mobility".

Exercise 4

a) 1   c) 3   e) 2   g) 2
b) 2   d) 1   f) 1

Exercise 5.1

1. Sickness   5. Contraction   9. Anemia
2. Pregnancy   6. Defect   10. Complication
3. Infection   7. Transfusion   11. Diabetes
4. Fracture   8. Absence   12. Allergy

Exercise 5.2

CONDITION	PRIMARY CODE	SECONDARY CODE
1. Uremic pericarditis	N18.8	I32.8
2. Gonococcal arthritis	A54.4	M01.3
3. Mumps meningitis	B26.1	G02.0
4. Tuberculous spondylitis	A18.0	M49.0
5. Gouty iritis	M10.9	H22.1

Exercise 6.1

1. T	3. T	5. F	7. F
2. T	4. F	6. T	8. T

Exercise 6.2

1. B	3. M	5. S	7. B	9. M
2. S	4. B	6. M	8. S	10. M

Exercise 6.3

I. a) The block entitled "Human immunodeficiency virus (HIV) disease.
   b) Codes within the block: B20 – B24.

II. Nutritional Anemias :   2, 5
   Hemolytic Anemias :   1, 4
   Aplastic Anemias: 6, 3

Exercise 6.4

1. F	3. T	5. F
2. F	4. F	6. F

Exercise 6.5

1. F	2. F	3. F	4. F	5. F

Exercise 6.6

1. Inflammation of *meninges* leads to meningitis
2. Myelitis refers to the *tissues* of the spinal cord
3. *Encephalitis* refers to the inflammation of brain tissue
4. Most dagger codes referred to in this chapter can be found in *Chapter I*
5. Central nervous system includes brain and *spinal cord*

Exercise 6.7

1. F	2. F	3. F	4. F	5. F

Exercise 6.8

1. T	2. T	3. F	4. F	5. T

Exercise 6.9

1. F   2. T   3. F   4. T   5. T

Exercise 6.10

1. U   3. U   5. U   7. U   9. L
2. L   4. L   6. L   8. U   10. L

Exercise 6.11

1. F   2. T   3. F   4. F   5. T

Exercise 6.12

1. F   2. T   3. F   4. T   5. F

Exercise 6.13

1. F   2. T   3. T   4. T   5. F

Exercise 6.14

Chapter XIV has *11* blocks, the first *six* of them are concerned with the urinary system: the next block covers the diseases of the *male* genital organs, the following block dealing with the disorders of breast, the next two blocks covering disorders of the female *genital* system; and the last block (*N99*) covering other disorders of the genitourinary system.

Exercise 6.15

Chapter XV has *8* blocks. The first 3 blocks are concerned with pregnancy, the next three blocks cover *delivery* and its complications; the following block covers the *puerparium* (including *lactation* problems), and the *last* block covers other conditions, which complicate *pregnancy* and childbirth.

Exercise 6.16

The perinatal period begins at *22* completed weeks (*154* days) of gestation (the time when birth weight is normally *500g*), and ends *seven* completed days after *birth.*

Exercise 6.17

1. T   2. T   3. F   4. T   5. F

Exercise 6.18

Signs and *Symptoms* pointing to a *definite* diagnosis will have been *assigned* to a category in the *appropriate* chapter.

Exercise 6.19

1. F   2. T   3. T   4. T   5. F

Exercise 6.20

The codes for external causes (*V01-Y89*) should be used together with a code from Chapter *XIX*. Causes of death should preferably be coded from both chapters: Chapter *XIX* and Chapter *XX*, but if only *one* code is tabulated then the code from Chapter *XX* should be used in preference.

Exercise 6.21

1. X	3. ✓	5. ✓	7. X	9. ✓
2. ✓	4. ✓	6. X	8. ✓	10. X

Exercise 6.22

The title of Chapter XXII is *Codes for Special Purposes*. It has been assigned a total of 100 codes (U00-U99). Codes U00-U49 are to be used for the *provisional* assignment of new diseases of uncertain *etiology*. Codes U50-*U99* may be used in *research*.

Exercise 7

1.   The main condition is the condition *diagnosed* at the *end* of the *episode* of health care, *primarily* responsible for the patient receiving treatment or being investigated.
2.   Other conditions are those conditions, which *coexist* or *develop* during the episode of health care and affect the *management* of the patient.
3.   According to Rule MB4 (specificity), if the diagnosis recorded as the "main condition" describes a condition in *general* terms, and a term that provides more *precise* information, reselect the *latter* as the "*main condition*".

Exercise 8

    1. (b)

    2. (c)

1. a) The responsibility for deciding on the logical sequence of death lies with the certifying *doctor*.

    b) In case of deaths due to injury, it is the ***External Cause*** code (Chapter *XX)* that should be used for single cause coding and tabulating underlying cause.

    c) The *asterisk* code should not be used for mortality coding. The dagger code is the ***primary*** code for this purpose.

    d) According to the General Principle when more than one condition is entered on the certificate, the condition entered alone on the *lowest* used line for Part I should be selected *only* if it could have given rise to all the conditions entered *above* it.

Exercise 9

The three main changes are:

    1. There are now three volumes in ICD-10.

    2. There are now 22 chapters.

    3. The structure of the code has changed.

CODING EXERCISES
(Chapters I – XXI)

CODING EXERCISE – CHAPTER I

I. Using Volume 3 (Index) of ICD-10, provide appropriate codes for the following diagnostic statements:

No.	Diagnostic statements	ICD-10 code
1	Paratyphoid fever, C	A01.3
2	Congenital Syphilis	A50.9
3	Falciparum malaria with cerebral complications	B50.0✝G94.8*
4	Ascariasis with intestinal complications	B77.0✝K93.8*
5	Salmonella enteritis	A02.0
6	Tuberculosis of lung	A16.2
7	Candidiasis of nails	B37.2
8	Sequelae of genitourinary tuberculosis	B90.1
9	Pediculosis capitis	B85.0
10	Streptococcal infection	A49.1
11	Taenia saginata infection	B68.1
12	Tetatnus neonatorum	A33
13	Tonsillar diphtheria	A36.0
14	Cholera	A00.9
15	Acute amebic dysentery	A06.0
16	Chronic viral hepatitis, type C	B18.2
17	Brucellosis due to Brucella canis	A23.3
18	Tuberculoid leprosy	A30.1
19	German measles	B06.9
20	Viral conjunctivitis	B30.9✝H13.1*

II. Using Volume 1 (Four-Character Categories, Tabular List), provide *complete* diagnostic statements for the following codes:

No	ICD-10 code	Diagnostic statement
1	A40.0	Septicemia due to streptococcus, group A
2	B05.4	Measles with intestinal complications
3	A36.9	Diphtheria, unspecified
4	B23.0	Acute HIV infection syndrome
5	A18.0✝	Tuberculosis of bones and joints

CODING EXERCISE – CHAPTER II

III.   Using Volume 3 (Index) of the ICD-10, provide appropriate codes for the following diagnostic statements:

No.	Diagnostic statements	ICD-10 code
1	Brain tumour, benign	D33.2
2	Skin cancer of uncertain behavior	D48.5
3	Bronchial carcinoma, secondary	C78.0
4	Malignant mass of face, primary	C76.0
5	Carcinoma of posterior stomach wall, secondary	C78.8
6	In situ neoplasm of internal auditory canal	D02.3
7	Malignant lump of inner ear, primary	C30.1
8·	Lung tumour of unknown behavior	D38.1
9	Benign neoplasm of cervix canal	D26.0
10	Neoplasm of lingual tonsil, benign	D10.1
11	Malignant neoplasm of nasal cavity, primary	C30.0
12	Uterine cancer of uncertain behavior	D39.0
13	In situ neoplasm of the skin of leg	D04.7
14	Benign neoplasm of ventral surface of tongue	D10.1
15	Malignant lump of vulva, secondary	C79.8
16	Malignant mass of chin, primary	C44.3
17	Neoplasm of upper gum, benign	D10.3
18	Breast tumor of uncertain behavior	D48.6
19	Benign neoplasm of bladder neck	D30.3
20	Carcinoma of wrist bone, secondary	C79.5

II. Using Volume 1 (Four-Character Categories, Tabular List), provide *complete* diagnostic statements for the following codes:

No.	ICD-10 code	Diagnostic statement
1	D48.6	Neoplasm of breast, uncertain behaviour
2	C25.9	Malignant neoplasm of pancreas, unspecified
3	D10.2	Benign neoplasm of floor of mouth
4	D06.0	Carcinoma in situ of endocervix
5	D30.3	Benign neoplasm of bladder

CODING EXERCISE – CHAPTER III

I.   Using Volume 3 (Index) of ICD-10, provide appropriate codes for the following diagnostic statements:

No.	Diagnostic statements	ICD-10 code
1	Hemophilia, type C	D68.1
2	Neutropenic splenomegaly	D70
3	Hereditary eosinophilia	D72.1
4	Drug induced nonautoimmune hemolytic anemia	D59.2
5	Von Willebrand disease	D68.0
6	Christmas disease	D67
7	Idiopathic thrombocytopenic purpura	D69.3
8	Constitutional aplastic anemia	D61.0
9	Chronic red cell aplasia	D60.0
10	Paroxysmal nocturnal hemoglobinuria	D59.4
11	Deficiency of factor XII	D68.2
12	Sickle-cell trait	D57.3
13	Iron deficiency anemia	D50.9
14	Vascular pseudohemophilia	D69.8
15	Agranulocytosis	D70
16	Abscess of spleen	D73.3
17	Gray platelet syndrome	D69.1
18	Congenital dysphagocytosis	D71
19	Sarcoidosis of lymph nodes and lung	D86.2
20	Vitamin B12 deficiency anemia	D51.9

II. Using Volume 1 (Four-character categories, Tabular List), provide *complete* diagnostic statements for the following codes:

No.	ICD-10 code	Diagnostic statement
1	D56.0	Alpha thalassaemia
2	D72.1	Eosinophilia
3	D57.0	Sickle-cell anaemia with crisis
4	D73.5	Infarction of spleen
5	D50.9	Iron deficiency anaemia, unspecified

CODING EXERCISE – CHAPTER IV

I. Using Volume 3 (Index) of the ICD-10, provide appropriate codes for the following diagnostic statement:

No.	Diagnostic statements	ICD-10 code
1	Insulin-dependent diabetes mellitus, with coma	E10.0
2	Drug-induced hypoglycemia with coma (nondiabetic)	E15
3	Drug-induced Cushing's syndrome	E24.2
4	Pituitary gigantism	E22.0
5	Marasmic kwashiorkor	E42
6	Third degree malnutrition	E43
7	Vitamin A deficiency with conjunctival xerosis	E50.0✝H13.8*
8	Obesity due to excess calories	E66.0
9	Classical phenylketonuria	E70.0
10	Non-insulin-dependent diabetes mellitus with ketoacidosis	E11.1
11	Hypercholesterolemia with Hyperglyceridemia	E78.2
12	Cystic fibrosis with intestinal manifestations	E84.1
13	Iron deficiency	E61.1
14	Hyperthyroidism with diffuse goiter	E05.0
15	Polycystic ovarian syndrome	E28.2
16	Non-insulin-dependent diabetes with unspecified complications	E11.8
17	Idiopathic hypoparathyroidism	E20.0
18	Thiamine deficiency with beriberi	E51.1
19	Lactose intolerance	E73.9
20	Insulin-dependent diabetes mellitus, with renal complications	E10.2

II. Using Volume I (Four-Character Categories, Tabular List), provide *complete* diagnostic statements for the following codes:

No.	ICD-10 code	Diagnostic statement
1	E84.1	Cystic fibrosis with intestinal manifestation
2	E87.4	Mixed disorders of acid-base balance
3	E10.4	Insulin-dependent diabetes with neurological Complications
4	E50.5	Vitamin A deficiency with night blindness
5	E11.9	Non-insulin dependent diabetes, without complications

CODING EXERCISE – CHAPTER V

I. Using Volume 3 (Index) of the ICD-10, provide appropriate codes for the following diagnostic statement:

No.	Diagnostic statements	ICD-10 code
1	Dementia of old age	F03
2	Anxiety disorder due to alcohol	F10.8
3	Obsessional rituals	F42.1
4	Dissociative sensory loss	F44.6
5	Undifferentiated somatoform disorder	F45.1
6	Atypical bulimia nervosa	F50.3
7	Hypochondrical disorder	F45.2
8	Anorexia nervosa	F50.0
9	Depersonalization – derealization syndrome	F48.1
10	Acute stress reaction	F43.0
11	Hyperkinetic disorder	F90.9
12	Excessive thumb-sucking in childhood	F98.8
13	Nocturnal psychogenic enuresis	F98.0
14	Developmental learning disorder	F81.9
15	Catatonic schizophrenia	F20.2
16	Delirium due to alcohol withdrawal	F10.4
17	Separation anxiety disorder of childhood	F93.0
18	Organic hallucinosis	F06.0
19	Bipolar affective disorder, unspecified	F31.9
20	Sibling rivalry disorder	F93.3

II. Using Volume 1 (Four-Character Categories, Tabular list), provide *complete* diagnostic statements for the following codes:

No.	ICD-10 code	Diagnostic statement
1	F30.2	Mania with psychotic symptoms
2	F50.2	Bulimia nervosa
3	F72.0	Severe mental retardation with no impairment of behaviour
4	F20.0	Paranoid schizophrenia
5	F41.1	Generalized anxiety disorder

CODING EXERCISE – CHAPTER VI

I. Using Volume 3 (Index) of the ICD-10, provide appropriate codes for the following diagnostic statement:

No.	Diagnostic statements	ICD-10 code
1	Migraine without aura	G43.0
2	Parkinson's disease	G20
3	Circumscribed brain atrophy	G31.0
4	Alzheimer's disease, late onset	G30.1
5	Drug-induced chorea	G25.4
6	Multiple sclerosis	G35
7	Epilepsy	G40.9
8	Cluster headache syndrome	G44.0
9	Sleep disorder	G47.9
10	Carpal tunnel syndrome	G56.0
11	Idiopathic progressive neuropathy	G60.3
12	Myasthenia gravis	G70.0
13	Muscular dystrophy	G71.0
14	Flaccid paraplegia	G82.0
15	Spastic hemiplegia	G81.1
16	Ataxic cerebral palsy	G80.4
17	Compression of brain	G93.5
18	Obstructive hydrocephalus	G91.1
19	Alcoholic myopathy	G72.1
20	Eaton-Lambert syndrome	C80✝G73.1*

II. Using Volume 1 (Four-Character Categories, Tabular List), provide *complete* diagnostic statements for the following codes:

No.	ICD-10 code	Diagnostic statement
1	G80.0	Spastic cerebral palsy
2	G00.2	Streptococcal meningitis
3	G20	Parkinson's disease
4	G30	Alzheimer's disease
5	G40.3	Generalized idiopathic epilepsy and epileptic syndromes

CODING EXERCISE – CHAPTER VII

I. Using Volume 3 (Index) of the ICD-10, provide appropriate codes for the following diagnostic statement:

No.	Diagnostic statements	ICD-10 code
1	Vertical strabismus	H50.2
2	Sudden visual loss	H53.1
3	Hypermetropia	H52.0
4	Hereditary choroidal dystrophy	H31.2
5	Hordeolum	H00.0
6	Chalazion	H00.1
7	Blepharitis	H01.0
8	Deformity of orbit	H05.3
9	Pterygium	H11.0
10	Corneal ulcer	H16.0
11	Keratitis	H16.9
12	Traumatic cataract	H26.1
13	Low-tension glaucoma	H40.1
14	Traction detachment of retina	H33.4
15	Vitreous hemorrhage	H43.1
16	Double vision	H53.2
17	Astigmatism	H52.2
18	Senile nuclear cataract	H25.1
19	Blindness, one eye	H54.4
20	Lens-induced iridocyclitis	H20.2

II. Using Volume 1 (Four-Character Categories, Tabular List), provide *complete* diagnostic statements for the following codes:

No.	ICD-10 code	Diagnostic statement
1	H54.0	Blindness, both eyes
2	H10.1	Acute atopic conjunctivitis
3	H26.3	Drug-induced cataract
4	H40.1	Primary open-angle glaucoma
5	H49.9	Paralytic strabismus unspecified

CODING EXERCISE – CHAPTER VIII

I. Using Volume 3 (Index) of the ICD-10, provide appropriate codes for the following diagnostic statement:

No.	Diagnostic statements	ICD-10 code
1	Tinnitus	H93.1
2	Otorrhea	H92.1
3	Conductive hearing loss, bilateral	H90.0
4	Disorder of eighth cranial nerve	H93.3
5	Sudden (idiopathic) deafness	H91.2
6	Polyp of middle ear	H74.4
7	Meniere's disease	H81.0
8	Acoustic trauma	H83.3
9	Cochlear otosclerosis	H80.2
10	Lermoyez' syndrome	H81.3
11	Eustachian salpingitis	H68.0
12	Acute mastoiditis	H70.0
13	Chronic myringitis	H73.1
14	Presbycusis	H91.1
15	Abscess of external ear	H60.0
16	Chronic mucoid otitis media	H65.3
17	Labyrinthine dysfunction	H83.2
18	Sensorineural hearing loss, bilateral	H90.3
19	Obstruction of Eustachian tube	H68.1
20	Perichondritis of external ear	H61.0

II. Using Volume 1 (Four-Character Categories, Tabular List), provide *complete* diagnostic statements for the following codes:

No.	ICD-10 code	Diagnostic statement
1	H66.0	Acute suppurative otitis media
2	H61.2	Impacted cerumen
3	H72.0	Central perforation of tympanic membrane
4	H81.1	Benign paroxysmal vertigo
5	H91.9	Hearing loss, unspecified

CODING EXERCISE – CHAPTER IX

I. Using Volume 3 (Index) of the ICD-10, provide appropriate codes
for the following diagnostic statement:

No.	Diagnostic statements	ICD-10 code
1	Atherosclerosis of aorta	I70.0
2	Raynaud's syndrome	I73.0
3	Rupture of artery	I77.2
4	Phlebitis of femoral vein	I80.1
5	External thrombosed hemorrhoids	I84.3
6	Varicose veins of lower extremities with ulcer	I83.0
7	Esophageal varices with bleeding	I85.0
8	Hypotension due to drugs	I95.2
9	Cardiac arrest	I46.9
10	Postcardiotomy syndrome	I97.0
11	Necrosis of artery	I77.5
12	Atherosclerosis of renal artery	I70.1
13	Moyamoya disease	I67.5
14	Cerebral infarction	I63.9
15	Cardiac septal defect, acquired	I51.0
16	Sick sinus syndrome	I49.5
17	Ventricular fibrillation	I49.0
18	Occlusion of vertebral artery	I65.0
19	Supraventricular tachycardia	I47.1
20	Sudden cardiac death	I46.1

II. Using Volume 1 (Four-Character Categories, Tabular List), provide
complete diagnostic statements for the following codes:

No.	ICD-10 code	Diagnostic statement
1	I11	Hypertensive heart disease
2	I20.0	Unstable angina
3	I50.1	Left ventricular failure
4	I72.0	Aneurysm of carotid artery
5	I05.9	Mitral valve disease, unspecified

I. Using Volume 3 (Index) of the ICD-10, provide appropriate codes for the following diagnostic statement:

No.	Diagnostic statements	ICD-10 code
1	Common cold	J00
2	Acute respiratory failure	J96.0
3	Streptococcal pharyngitis	J02.0
4	Acute maxillary sinusitis	J01.0
5	Fibrothorax	J94.1
6	Nonallergic asthma	J45.1
7	Pneumoconiosis due to talc dust	J62.0
8	Viral pneumonia with influenza	J11.0
9	Chronic pneumothorax	J93.8
10	Chronic obstructive pulmonary disease	J44.9
11	MacLeod's syndrome	J43.0
12	Simple chronic bronchitis	J41.0
13	Chronic laryngitis	J37.0
14	Chronic disease of tonsils and adenoids	J35.9
15	Polyp of nasal cavity	J33.0
16	Allergic rhinitis due to pollen	J30.1
17	Pneumonia due to pseudomonas	J15.1
18	Acute bronchiolitis	J21.9
19	Stenosis of larynx	J38.6
20	Centrilobular emphysema	J43.2

II. Using Volume 1 (Four-Character Categories, Tabular List), provide *complete* diagnostic statements for the following codes:

No.	ICD-10 code	Diagnostic statement
1	J20.6	Acute bronchitis due to rhinovirus
2	J60	Coalworker's pneumoconiosis
3	J34.2	Deviated nasal septum
4	J85.1	Abscess of lung with pneumonia
5	J03.0	Streptococcal tonsillitis

CODING EXERCISE – CHAPTER XI

I. Using Volume 3 (Index) of the ICD-10, provide appropriate codes for the following diagnostic statement:

No.	Diagnostic statements	ICD-10 code
1	Toxic liver disease with acute hepatitis	K71.2
2	Cyst of pancreas	K86.2
3	Gastrointestinal hemorrhage	K92.2
4	Celiac disease	K90.0
5	Hernia with gangrene and obstruction	K46.1
6	Postoperative intestinal obstruction	K91.3
7	Acute pancreatitis	K85
8	Acute gastric ulcer with perforation	K25.1
9	Alcoholic gastritis	K29.2
10	Atrophy of tongue papillae	K14.4
11	Vesicular stomatitis	K12.1
12	Chronic gingivitis	K05.1
13	Abrasion of teeth	K03.1
14	Teething syndrome	K00.7
15	Radicular cyst	K04.8
16	Gingival recession	K06.0
17	Acute appendicitis with generalized peritonitis	K35.0
18	Crohn's disease of large intestine	K50.1
19	Anorectal fistula	K60.5
20	Functional diarrhea	K59.1

II. Using Volume 1 (Four-Character Categories, Tabular List), provide *complete* diagnostic statements for the following codes:

No.	ICD-10 code	Diagnostic statement
1	K26.0	Acute duodenal ulcer with hemorrhage
2	K35.1	Acute appendicitis with peritoneal abscess
3	K41.1	Bilateral femoral hernia, with gangrene
4	K28.5	Chronic gastrojejunal ulcer with perforation
5	K72.1	Chronic hepatic failure

CODING EXERCISE – CHAPTER XII

I. Using Volume 3 (Index) of the ICD-10, provide appropriate codes for the following diagnostic statement:

No.	Diagnostic statements	ICD-10 code
1	Vitiligo	L80
2	Decubitus ulcer	L89
3	Acne tropica	L70.3
4	Mucinosis of skin	L98.5
5	Xerosis cutis	L85.3
6	Localized hypertrichosis	L68.2
7	Alopecia universalis	L63.1
8	Solar urticaria	L56.3
9	Lichen planus	L43.9
10	Psoriasis vulgaris	L40.0
11	Pruritis vulvae	L29.2
12	Seborrhea capitis	L21.0
13	Bullous pemphigoid	L12.0
14	Cellulitis of finger	L03.0
15	Onychogryphosis	L60.2
16	Acute radiodermatitis	L58.0
17	Linear scleroderma	L94.1
18	Keloid scar	L91.0
19	Bockhart's impetigo	L01.0
20	Pemphigus vegetans	L10.1

II. Using Volume 1 (Four-Character Categories, Tabular List), provide *complete* diagnostic statements for the following codes:

No.	ICD-10 code	Diagnostic statement
1	L70.0	Acne vulgaris
2	L60.0	Ingrowing nail
3	L50.6	Contact urticaria
4	L40.1	Generalized pustular psoriasis
5	L03.2	Cellulitis of face

CODING EXERCISE – CHAPTER XIII

I. Using Volume 3 (Index) of the ICD-10, provide appropriate codes for the following diagnostic statement:

No.	Diagnostic statements	ICD-10 code
1	Juvenile rheumatoid arthritis	M08.0
2	Flat foot, acquired	M21.4
3	Postural kyphosis	M40.0
4	Infantile idiopathic scoliosis	M41.0
5	Adult osteochondrosis of spine	M42.1
6	Spinal stenosis	M48.0
7	Pott's curvature	A18.0✝M49.0*
8	Infective myositis	M60.0
9	Low back pain	M54.5
10	Calcific tendonitis	M65.2
11	Contracture of muscle	M62.4
12	Muscle strain	M62.6
13	Prepatellar bursitis	M70.2
14	Rupture of synovium	M66.1
15	Achilles tendonitis	M76.6
16	Osteoporosis of disuse	M81.2
17	Senile osteomalacia	M83.1
18	Acquired deformity of nose	M95.0
19	Reiter's disease	M02.3
20	Gout due to renal impairment	M10.3

II. Using Volume 1 (Four-Character Categories, Tabular List), provide *complete* diagnostic statements for the following codes:

No.	ICD-10 code	Diagnostic statement
1	M45	Ankylosing spondylitis
2	M70.1	Bursitis of hand
3	M81.0	Postmenopausal osteoporosis
4	M06.9	Rheumatoid arthritis, unspecified
5	M86.2	Subacute osteomyelitis

I. Using Volume 3 (Index) of the ICD-10, provide appropriate codes for the following diagnostic statement:

No.	Diagnostic statements	ICD-10 code
1	Inversion of uterus	N85.5
2	Chronic obstructive pyelonephritis	N11.1
3	Acute renal failure with medullary necrosis	N17.2
4	Primary amenorrhea	N91.0
5	Female sterility associated with anovulation	N97.0
6	Post procedural renal failure	N99.0
7	Endometriosis of uterus	N80.0
8	Acute vaginitis	N76.0
9	Cyst of Bartholin's gland	N75.0
10	Atrophy of prostate	N42.2
11	Impotence of organic origin	N48.4
12	Infected hydrocele	N43.1
13	Atrophy of breast	N64.2
14	Chronic salpingitis	N70.1
15	Male sterility	N46
16	Polyp of vulva	N84.3
17	Primary oligomenorrhea	N91.3
18	Premenstrual tension syndrome	N94.3
19	Nonspecific urethritis	N34.1
20	Stress incontinence	N39.3

II. Using Volume 1 (Four-Character Categories, Tabular List), provide *complete* diagnostic statements for the following codes:

No.	ICD-10 code	Diagnostic statement
1	N71.0	Acute inflammatory disease of uterus
2	N80.1	Endometriosis of ovary
3	N97.1	Female infertility of tubal origin
4	N17.0	Acute renal failure with tubular necrosis
5	N40	Hyperplasia of prostate

CODING EXERCISE – CHAPTER XV

I. Using Volume 3 (Index) of the ICD-10, provide appropriate codes for the following diagnostic statement:

No.	Diagnostic statements	ICD-10 code
1	Spontaneous breech delivery	O80.1
2	Missed abortion	O02.1
3	Multiple pregnancy	O30.9
4	Malformation of placenta	O43.1
5	Pre-term delivery	O60
6	Obstructed labor due to locked twins	O66.1
7	Postpartum coagulation defects	O72.3
8	Infection of obstetric surgical wound	O86.0
9	Maternal care for cervical incompetence	O34.3
10	Delivery by emergency cesarean section	O82.1
11	Antepartum hemorrhage with coagulation defect	O46.0
12	Placenta previa without hemorrhage	O44.0
13	Threatened abortion	O20.0
14	Hemorrhoids in pregnancy	O22.4
15	Infections of bladder in pregnancy	O23.1
16	Low forceps delivery	O81.0
17	Pyrexia during labor	O75.2
18	Galactorrhea	O92.6
19	Anemia complicating pregnancy	O99.0
20	Abdominal pregnancy	O00.0

II. Using Volume 1 (Four-Character Categories, Tabular List), provide *complete* diagnostic statements for the following codes:

No.	ICD-10 code	Diagnostic statement
1	O69.0	Labour and delivery complicated by prolapse of cord
2	O91.1	Abscess of breast associated with childbirth
3	O15.1	Eclampsia in labour
4	O04.2	Incomplete medical abortion, complicated by embolism
5	O03.9	Complete spontaneous abortion, without complication

I. Using Volume 3 (Index) of the ICD-10, provide appropriate codes for the following diagnostic statement:

No.	Diagnostic statements	ICD-10 code
1	Fetal death	P95
2	Meconium plug syndrome	P76.0
3	Noninfective neonatal diarrhea	P78.3
4	Coma of the newborn	P91.5
5	Umbilical polyp of newborn	P83.6
6	Dehydration of newborn	P74.1
7	Urinary tract infection of the newborn	P39.3
8	Respiratory failure of newborn	P28.5
9	Cold injury syndrome	P80.0
10	Aspiration of blood from newborn	P24.2
11	Congenital pneumonia due to pseudomonas	P23.5
12	Intrauterine hypoxia	P20.9
13	Birth injury to spleen	P15.1
14	Sepsis of newborn due to streptococcus, group B	P36.0
15	Fetal blood loss from placenta	P50.2
16	Neonatal hematemesis	P54.0
17	ABO isoimmunization of fetus and newborn	P55.1
18	Hydrops fetalis due to isoimmunization	P56.0
19	Neonatal jaundice due to polycythemia	P58.3
20	Kernicterus due to isoimmunization	P57.0

II. Using Volume 1 (Four-Character Categories, Tabular List), provide *complete* diagnostic statements for the following codes:

No.	ICD-10 code	Diagnostic statement
1	P07.2	Extreme immaturity
2	P37.5	Neonatal candidiasis
3	P00.5	Fetus and newborn affected by maternal injury
4	P22.0	Respiratory distress syndrome of newborn
5	P90	Convulsions of newborn

CODING EXERCISE – CHAPTER XVII

I. Using Volume 3 (Index) of the ICD-10, provide appropriate codes
for the following diagnostic statement:

No.	Diagnostic statements	ICD-10 code
1	Down's syndrome	Q90.9
2	Fragile X chromosome	Q99.2
3	Spina bifida occulta	Q76.0
4	Osteogenesis imperfecta	Q78.0
5	Xeroderma pigmentosum	Q82.1
6	Conjoined twins	Q89.4
7	Klinefelter's syndrome	Q98.4
8	Congenital deformity of knee	Q68.2
9	Renal dysplasia	Q61.4
10	Displacement of ureter	Q62.6
11	Marfan's syndrome	Q87.4
12	Undescended testicle, unilateral	Q53.1
13	Perineal hypospadias	Q54.3
14	Atresia of bile ducts	Q44.2
15	Cleft lip, unilateral	Q36.9
16	Web of larynx	Q31.0
17	Ventricular septal defect	Q21.0
18	Tetralogy of Fallot	Q21.3
19	Arnold-Chiari syndrome	Q07.0
20	Patent ductus arteriosus	Q25.0

II. Using Volume 1 (Four-Character Categories, Tabular List), provide
complete diagnostic statements for the following codes:

No.	ICD-10 code	Diagnostic statement
1	Q35.1	Cleft hard palate
2	Q03.8	Other congenital hydrocephalus
3	Q98.0	Klinefelter's syndrome karyotype 47, XXY
4	Q13.3	Congenital corneal opacity
5	Q65.1	Congenital dislocation of hip, bilateral

CODING EXERCISE – CHAPTER XVIII

I. Using Volume 3 (Index) of the ICD-10, provide appropriate codes for the following diagnostic statements:

No.	Diagnostic statements	ICD-10 code
1	Restlessness	R45.1
2	Persistent fever	R50.1
3	Headache	R51
4	Chronic intractable pain	R52.1
5	Febrile convulsions	R56.0
6	Lymphadenopathy	R59.1
7	Abnormal weight loss	R63.4
8	Ataxic gait	R26.0
9	Meningismus	R29.1
10	Painful urination	R30.9
11	Finding of cocaine in blood	R78.2
12	Abnormality of red blood cells	R71
13	Isolated proteinuria	R80
14	Abnormal glucose tolerance test	R73.0
15	Unattended death	R98
16	Glycosuria	R81
17	Generalized edema	R60.1
18	Hypovolemic shock	R57.1
19	Auditory hallucination	R44.0
20	Extrarenal uremia	R39.2

II. Using Volume 1 (Four-Character Categories, TABULAR LIST), provide *complete* diagnostic statements for the following codes:

No.	ICD-10 code	Diagnostic statement
1	R95	Sudden infant death syndrome
2	R59.0	Localized enlarged lymph nodes
3	R46.0	Very low level of personal hygiene
4	R94.4	Abnormal results of kidney function studies
5	R04.1	Haemorrhage from throat

CODING EXERCISE – CHAPTER XIX

I. Using Volume 3 (Index) of the ICD-10, provide appropriate codes for the following diagnostic statement:

No.	Diagnostic statements	ICD-10 code
1	Open wound of knee	S81.0
2	Dislocation of hip	S73.0
3	Crushing injury of hip with thigh	S77.2
4	Heat exhaustion	T67.5
5	Psychological abuse	T74.3
6	Traumatic shock	T79.4
7	Rh incompatibility reaction	T80.4
8	Injury of popliteal vein	S85.5
9	Contusion of knee	S80.0
10	Open wound of abdominal wall	S31.1
11	Burn of third degree of wrist and hand	T23.3
12	Frostbite with tissue necrosis of neck	T34.1
13	Poisoning by sulfonamides	T37.0
14	Epidural hemorrhage	S06.4
15	Concussion	S06.0
16	Burns involving 50-59% of unspecified site of body surface	T31.5
17	Superficial frostbite of arm	T33.4
18	Poisoning by local anesthetics	T41.3
19	Toxic effect of hydrogen sulfide	T59.6
20	Motion sickness	T75.3

II. Using Volume 1 (Four-Character Categories, Tabular List), provide *complete* diagnostic statements for the following codes:

No.	ICD-10 code	Diagnostic statement
1	S22.3	Fracture of rib
2	T53.1	Toxic effect of chloroform
3	T17.4	Foreign body in trachea
4	T01.0	Open wounds involving head with neck
5	T65.2	Toxic effect of tobacco and nicotine

CODING EXERCISE – CHAPTER XX

I. Using Volume 1 and Volume 3 (Index) of the ICD-10, provide appropriate codes for the following diagnostic statements:

NOTE: Use "Place of Occurrence" code at the fourth-character level for these accidents.

No.	Diagnostic statement	ICD-10 code
1	Exposure to X-ray radiation, in hospital	W88.2
2	Strangulation by pillow, in hotel	W75.5
3	Victim of volcanic eruption, at mountain	X35.8
4	Bitten by dog, on road	W54.4
5	War operations involving land mine explosion	Y36.2
6	Car accident	V49.9
7	Burn by hotplate, at home	X15.0
8	Legal intervention involving gas	Y35.2
9	Run over by machinery, at farm	W31.7
10	Choked on bone, at restaurant	W79.5
11	Cutting misadventure during heart catheterization	Y60.5
12	Asphyxia from forest fire	X09.8
13	Obstruction of esophagus by vomitus, home	W44.0
14	Collapse of burning building, at factory	X00.6
15	Drowning in bathtub, at home	W65.0
16	Motion sickness, at motorway	X51.4
17	Intentional self-harm by sleeping pills	X61.9
18	Mismatched blood in transfusion	Y65.0
19	Accidental poisoning by lead acetate	X44.9
20	Adverse effect of penicillin in therapeutic use	Y40.0

II. Using Volume 1 (Four-Character Categories, Tabular List), provide *complete* diagnostic statements for the following codes:

No.	ICD-10 code	Diagnostic statement
1	V87.3	Person injured in collision between car and bus (traffic)
2	W05.2	Fall involving wheelchair, in hospital
3	W53.0	Bitten by rat, at home
4	X72.9	Intentional self harm by handgun discharge
5	X45.9	Accidental poisoning by and exposure to alcohol

CODING EXERCISE – CHAPTER XXI

I. Using Volume 3 (Index) of the ICD-10, provide appropriate codes for the following diagnostic statement:

No.	Diagnostic statement	ICD-10 code
1	Supervision of normal first pregnancy	Z34.0
2	Prophylactic vaccination against smallpox	Z25.8
3	Carrier of viral hepatitis	Z22.5
4	Screening for neoplasm of breast	Z12.3
5	Laboratory examination	Z01.7
6	Observation for suspected tuberculosis	Z03.0
7	Contraceptive management	Z30.9
8	Genetic counseling	Z31.5
9	Personal history of allergy to penicillin	Z88.0
10	Family history of diabetes mellitus	Z83.3
11	Acquired absence of foot and ankle	Z89.4
12	Occupational health examination	Z10.0
13	Issue of medical certificate	Z02.7
14	Confirmed pregnancy	Z32.1
15	Follow-up examination following psychotherapy	Z09.3
16	Medical examination for driving license	Z02.4
17	Fertility test	Z31.4
18	Fitting of external breast prosthesis	Z44.3
19	Insertion of intrauterine contraceptive device	Z30.1
20	Medical examination for insurance purposes	Z02.6

II. Using Volume 1 (Four-Character Categories, Tabular List), provide *complete* diagnostic statements for the following codes:

No.	ICD-10 code	Diagnostic statement
1	Z94.5	Skin transplant status
2	Z01.2	Dental examination
3	Z99.3	Dependence on wheelchair
4	Z00.1	Routine child health examination
5	Z35.9	Supervision of high-risk pregnancy, unspecified

BIBLIOGRAPHY

BIBLIOGRAPHY

1. Ashley, J.S.A. Present state of statistics from hospital in-patient data and their uses. *British Journal of Preventive and Social Medicine.* 1972, 26, 135

2. Bain, D., Basset, W., and Haines, A. Difficulties encountered in classifying illness in general practice. *Journal of Royal College of General Practitioners.* 23, 474

3. Bertillon J. Classification of the causes of death (abstract). In: Transactions of the 15th International Congress on Hygiene Demography. Washington, 1912.

4. *Bulletin of the .Institute of International Statistics.* 1900, 12: 280. International list of causes of death. The Hague, International Statistical Institute, 1940.

5. Crombie, D.L. The nature of information in clinical decision-making. *Journal of Royal College of General Practitioners.* 1976, 5, 35-40.

6. Greenwood, M. *Medical statistics from Graunt to Farr.* Cambridge, Cambridge University Press, 1948.

7. *International classification of diseases for oncology* (ICD-0), second ed. Geneva, World Health Organization, 1990.

8. *International classification of impairments,* disabilities, and *handicaps. A manual of classification relating to the consequences of disease.* Geneva, World Health Organization, 1980.

9. *International classification of procedures in medicine* (ICPM). Vols. 1 and 2. Geneva, World Health Organization, 1978.

10. *International Nomenclature of Diseases.* Geneva, Council for International Organizations of Medical Sciences and World Health Organization.

11. Knibbs, G.H. The International Classification of Disease and Causes of Death and its revision. *Medical Journal of Australia*, 1929, 1:2-12.

12. Langmuir A. D. William Farr: founder of modern concepts of surveillance. *International Journal of Epidemiology*, 1976, 5, 13-18.

13. *Manual of the international statistical classification of diseases, injuries, and causes of death. Sixth Revision.* Geneva, World Health Organization, 1949.

14. *Manual of the international statistical classification of diseases, injuries, and causes of death.* Seventh Revision. Geneva, World Health Organization, 1958.

15. *Manual of the international statistical classification of disease, injuries, and causes of death.* Eight Revision. Geneva, World Health Organization, 1967.

16. *Manual of the international statistical classification of disease, injuries, and cause of death.* Ninth Revision. Geneva, World Health Organization, 1977.

17. *Manual of tumor nomenclature and coding* (MOTNAC). New York, American Cancer Society, 1968.

18. *Systematized nomenclature of medicine* (SNOMED). Chicago, College of American Pathologists, 1976.

19. *Systematized nomenclature of pathology* (SNOP). Chicago, College of American Pathologists, 1965.

20. *The ICD-10 classification of mental and behavioural disorders: clinical descriptions and diagnostic guidelines.* Geneva, World Health Organization, 1992.

INDEX